D0484946

BACKACHE

51 Ways to Relieve the Pain

Charles B. Inlander
and
Porter Shimer

A *People's Medical Society Book*

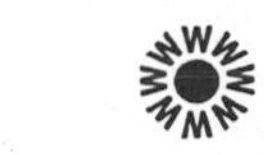

WALKER AND COMPANY
NEW YORK

Copyright © 1997 by People's Medical Society

A note to the reader: The ideas, procedures, and suggestions contained in this book are not intended as a substitute for consulting with your practitioner. All matters regarding your health require medical supervision.

All rights reserved. No part of this book may be reproduced or transmitted in any form or by any means, electronic or mechanical, including photocopying, recording, or by any information storage and retrieval system, without permission in writing from the Publisher.

First published in the United States of America in 1997
by Walker Publishing Company, Inc.

Published simultaneously in Canada by
Thomas Allen & Son Canada, Limited, Markham, Ontario

Library of Congress Cataloging-in-Publication Data

Inlander, Charles B.
Backache : 51 ways to relieve the pain /
Charles B. Inlander and Porter Shimer.
p. cm.
"A People's Medical Society book."
Includes index.
ISBN 0-8027-7516-0 (pbk.)
1. Backache–Popular works. I. Shimer, Porter. II. Title.
RD771.B217I54 1997
617.5'64–dc21

97-991
CIP

Printed in the United States of America

2 4 6 8 10 9 7 5 3 1

BACKACHE

■

Other Walker and Company Books
From the People's Medical Society

77 Ways to Beat Colds and Flu

■

67 Ways to Good Sleep

■

Headaches: 47 Ways to Stop the Pain

■

Stress: 63 Ways to Relieve Tension and Stay Healthy

CONTENTS

INTRODUCTION

Almost everyone I know suffers from backache. It's not because I'm in the midst of middle age. Most of my friends have complained about bad backs since their early 20s. In fact, backache seems to have become a national malady, a condition almost none of us can avoid or do too much about. Or can we?

Actually, there is a lot we can do about backache and its causes. Not only are there many effective ways to ease the pain of backache, but preventing recurring backache is possible, as well. If we take a "back-smart" approach to our lives, we can make back pain a rare and less devastating condition.

And that is why we have written this book. *Backache: 51 Ways to Relieve the Pain* is your complete guide to backache treatment and prevention.

Recognizing what can go wrong, and why your back hurts, is the first strategy to employ. In these pages, we explain your back and the problems that can arise. And if your sore back is making you suffer? *Backache: 51 Ways to Relieve the Pain* explains many tested and proven ways to ease the pain and become active and productive again. We also tell you what you need to know to prevent backache from striking twice. If you follow those tips, you'll drastically reduce the chances that your back will hurt again.

So what makes this book different from all those other books on backache? Plenty! First, this is not a book of opinions. The tips you will read in the pages that follow come from medical studies and reports. These are the strategies and techniques that are documented to work. While not all of these remedies will help everyone, we're confident that no matter what your back problem, there is important information in this book that will help you deal with the pain.

What also makes this book different is that it's easy to use and understand. It is written with you in mind, and we know that you want answers and relief. That's why vital information starts coming on the very first page and doesn't stop until you've finished the book.

As the nation's largest nonprofit consumer health advocacy organization, the People's Medical Society is committed to helping you get the information you need to take charge of your health and live an active and productive life. We're convinced that *Backache: 51 Ways to Relieve the Pain* will be an indispensable part of your health-care library.

Charles B. Inlander, President
People's Medical Society

BACKACHE

■

1 Understanding Backache

If it seems that just about everybody you talk with suffers from back pain of some type, it's because just about everybody does. "Anyone who lives an average life span without suffering from backache belongs to a privileged minority," says Hamilton Hall, M.D., orthopedic surgeon and founder of the Canadian Back Institute in Toronto, in his book *The Back Doctor.**

The rest of us 80 percent, in fact can expect to suffer from some form of back pain in our lifetimes. Recent studies and surveys report that approximately half of us who are of working age will suffer from backache in the coming year, and on any given day, a whopping 6.5 million people are too incapacitated by back pain to even get out of bed. One government survey has found that back pain is now the number-one reason people see their primary-care doctors, and other research shows that it's now second only to the common cold at causing us to miss work.

Recent sources also report that the financial strain of back pain is significant. Approximately 5 million Americans currently are partially disabled because of back pain, and another 2 million can't work at all. This accounts for 93 million lost workdays annually and approximately $10 billion in claims made for workers' compensation. When all costs are tallied, we lose, by some estimates, upward of $70 billion to our aching backs every year.

---

* Toronto: McClelland and Stewart, 1987.

What's more, the prevalence of back trouble is on the rise. "Throughout the medical profession, we are finding a shocking increase in both the frequency and severity of back problems," write Alfred O. Bonati, M.D., director and chief surgeon of the Gulf Coast Orthopedic Center Institute for Special Surgery in Hudson, Florida, and Shirley Linde, Ph.D., in their book *No More Back Pain*.*

The Origins of Back Pain

Why should such a vital part of the body be so vulnerable to aches and pains?

"The bottom line is that the human spine is poorly designed for a two-legged creature," say Richard Fraser, M.D., professor of neurosurgery at Cornell University Medical College, and Ann Forer in their book *The Well-Informed Patient's Guide to Back Surgery*.† "If we were still walking around on all fours, we might have fewer difficulties with our backs." Virtually all of our most common types of backache result from problems caused by gravity's downward pressure on the spine created by our upright posture, Fraser and Forer say.

This is not to say that we do not sorely mistreat our backs as well. Our all-too-civilized lifestyle is anything but civil to our backbones. According to one widely cited statistic, as many as 90 percent of our back problems have been estimated to have their roots in our lifestyle. For example, sitting subjects spinal discs to 50 percent more pressure than standing. Sitting done in a slouching manner can be even more stressful than lifting. Worse yet, our inactive lifestyles predispose us to weight gain, giving our spines a heavier burden to support. At the same time, inactivity weakens the muscles that could help the spine carry the added weight. "The sudden attack that seems to happen for no reason usually is caused by damage incurred gradually during the course of our lifetimes," Fraser and Forer say.

To understand backache, it's helpful to understand the back—especially since its complexity is one of the primary reasons backache is so common. With so many parts, so much can go wrong.

If the spine were merely one singular bone, as the term "backbone" implies, our troubles would be comparatively few. But the human

---

* New York: Pharos, 1991.

† New York: Dell, 1992.

spine is an anatomical marvel consisting of 24 separate bones called vertebrae (the top 7 are known as cervical vertebrae, the 12 in the midback are known as thoracic vertebrae, and the 5 in the lower back are called lumbar vertebrae). In addition, 23 spinal discs provide cushion devices between these vertebrae; 23 joints, called facet joints, keep these vertebrae interlocked and functioning as a singular unit;

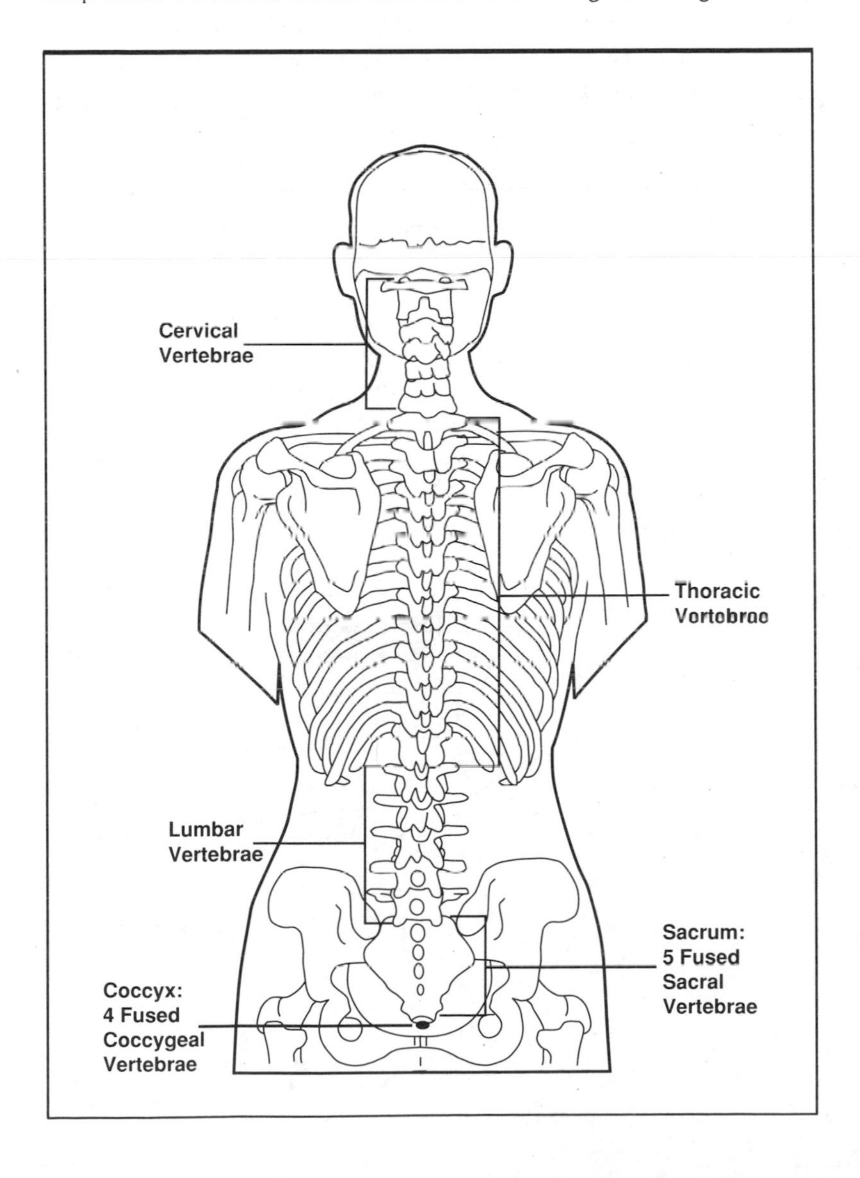

31 paired sets of nerves branch out from the spinal cord through small openings in the vertebrae; and 140 muscles work along with hundreds of ligaments and tendons to allow this stack of vertebrae to do more than just stand there.

Malfunctions of the vertebrae, discs, facet joints, nerves, or muscles can cause pain, singly or in combination. One source of pain can create other sources, producing a domino effect that can make the primary cause of back pain difficult to diagnose. No two back problems are identical. In fact, in most cases, back pain is idiopathic, meaning that no single, clear-cut cause is ever found.

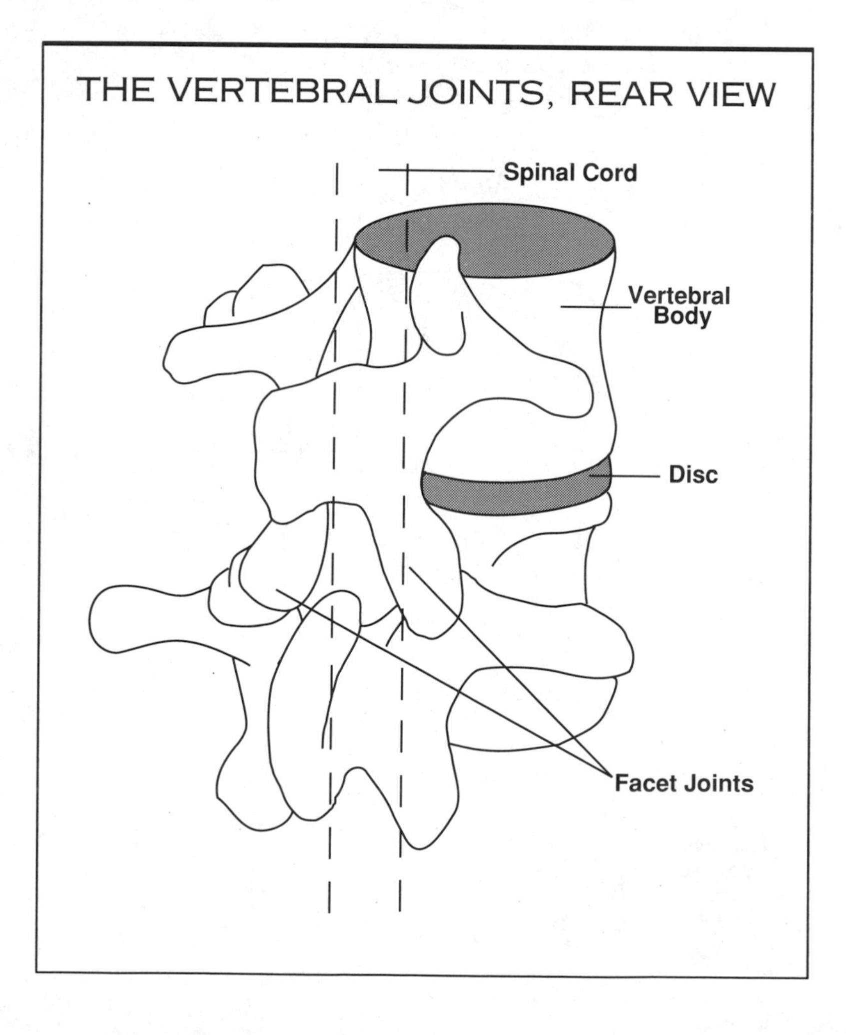

Yet most backaches respond well to treatment and self-care—even when the precise reason for the pain cannot be discovered. As Augustus A. White III, M.D., professor of orthopedic surgery at Harvard Medical School, humbly concedes in his book *Your Aching Back*, "We doctors are actually better at managing back problems than we are at finding their exact cause."*

Our backs are problematic, but they also are highly receptive to appropriate corrective measures when they do go on the blink.

What Can Go Wrong

Now that you have a basic idea of how your back is put together, let's take a closer look at how it can break down. As highly individual as back pain can be, most cases—80 percent, in fact, according to Hall—can be attributed to problems within one or more of the following three areas: the muscles of the back, its facet joints, and its discs.

Muscular Backache

This is by far the most common type of back pain and, fortunately, the least serious. If your back is hurting simply because you've strained a muscle by overexerting yourself and there isn't a more serious underlying problem, you'll feel a dull ache within about 24 hours of the overexertion. Complete relief usually comes within several days if the injured muscle is properly rested. (For tips on treatment, see Chapter 2.)

But muscular backache also can be the result of a spasm, a sudden, painful contraction of the muscles. Spasms, experienced as sharper, more knifelike pain, can be triggered by simple overexertion, but usually they're due to more complicated matters such as a worn facet joint or a problem with a spinal disc. The spasm is the body's way of immobilizing the injured area to prevent further harm: Muscles knot up to cause a kind of natural splint that, in addition to protecting the injured area locally, prevents further damage by causing pain so severe you don't feel like moving. If your muscular backache is being caused by a spasm, you'll know right away by the piercing pain. Your back also will feel exceptionally stiff, and the affected muscle (or muscles) will feel hard and knotty and will hurt more when probed.

---

* New York: Simon and Schuster, 1990.

Backache Due to a Faulty Facet Joint

Facet joints, the interlocking bones at the rear of the spine, can cause pain if the surrounding muscles are sprained (torn) or strained (stretched too far), perhaps by a sudden jerk or twist. They can also cause pain if the bones become worn due to arthritis or gradual wear and tear occurring naturally with aging, or if the discs that cushion them break down, causing friction as the joint becomes unnaturally compressed. This degeneration irritates the joint's sensitive linings, which consist of nerve-rich cartilage and a lubricating substance called synovial fluid. Facet joint problems also can trigger muscular backache by sending nearby muscles into painful spasm to immobilize the area.

Because facet joint injury may result in muscular backache, it may be difficult to tell which type of injury you're dealing with. Whereas exertion (an entire afternoon weeding the garden, for example) brings on muscular backache, events as minor as bending over or laughing too heartily can ignite back pain due to a worn facet joint. Shooting pain, called sciatica because it's caused by pressure on the sciatic nerve, which runs from the spine down the back of the leg, is also a sign of facet joint troubles. It usually will be felt in the buttocks and thighs as well as in the back. Another sign of facet joint injury: Back pain will worsen if you try to straighten up and subside if you lean forward.

Backache Due to a Bulging or Herniated Spinal Disc

Spinal discs are flat, round structures that consist of a tough outer ring of fibrous tissue surrounding a gelatinous center. These cushioning spinal discs are the spine's shock absorbers, and they can wear out. If, because of excessive wear, a disc begins to slip out of its place between the vertebrae, causing a bulge, it can cause pain by irritating nerves within the disc's outer shell. But if the disc herniates, or ruptures, the resulting protrusion can press on a nerve of the spinal cord or even on the spinal cord itself. This can produce excruciating pain felt locally as well as in the areas of the body serviced by the nerve being impinged—for example, the legs or the feet. In some cases, a piece of the ruptured disc can break free and lodge painfully against a

(continued on page 10)

LESS COMMON CAUSES OF BACK PAIN

There are other sources of back pain in addition to the three most common ones described in this chapter. Remember that 90 percent of all backaches are due to lifestyle factors and can be treated with self-care, so the odds are in your favor that you are not in the throes of a serious medical condition. If you are diagnosed with one of the following less common conditions, talk with your doctor about how to incorporate the tips in this book into your treatment program. Though your condition may not disappear on its own, self care and prevention can go a long way toward speeding your recovery or preventing a worsening or relapse.

■ **Ankylosing spondylitis.** This is a rare and potentially crippling form of arthritis in which vertebrae of the spine become fused due to the formation of bony growths, limiting movement and, in some cases, restricting breathing. In some cases, the disease develops rapidly, starting in the lower spine and spreading upward, while in others it affects the lower spine only. It has no known cure, though specific exercises done in the early stages of the disease can retard its development.

■ **Fractures.** Fractures in the spine's vertebrae can result from severe trauma such as a car accident or bad fall, but they also can be caused by a weakening of the vertebrae due to osteoporosis (see next page). Pain can result as muscles in the vicinity of the fracture go into spasm to help immobilize the injured area, but this pain usually subsides when the fracture heals. Fractures do not always cause pain, and some may heal on their own without treatment.

■ **Hyperlordosis and hyperkyphosis.** In these conditions, the natural curves of the spine become exaggerated to the point of putting undue pressure on facet joints and spinal discs. Hyperlordosis occurs when the forward tilt of the lower back becomes exaggerated, and hyperkyphosis results when the back-

(continued on next page)

(continued)

ward tilt of the upper back becomes exaggerated. A defect at birth can cause each of these excessive curves, as can osteoporosis (see below), muscle spasms, spinal fractures, and even bad posture due to pregnancy, obesity, or excessive wearing of high-heeled shoes. Treatment varies according to the condition and may include immobilizing the spine with a brace or performing surgery.

■ **Infections.** Infections of the spine are rare, but they can occur, due either to bacteria entering the body through an open wound in the area of the back or to a systemic disease such as tuberculosis, a urinary tract infection, an infection of the kidneys, or an infection of the sheath that covers the spinal cord (meningitis). Usually, a fever, headache, and other bodily discomforts, along with pain in the area of the back, will accompany such infections, which can be treated with antibiotics.

■ **Osteoarthritis.** Osteoarthritis is a disease in which joints become painfully inflamed. The cartilage within the joints may deteriorate and cause inflammation, or the lubricating substance (called synovial fluid) or the delicate membrane (called the synovial membrane) within the joints may become irritated. With regard to back pain, this inflammation usually occurs within the facet joints of the vertebrae, causing pain and stiffness that tend to be most severe after periods of inactivity (getting up in the morning can be especially uncomfortable) or when the weather is cold or damp. Osteoarthritis occurs in some form in almost everyone over age 60. This chronic condition can be controlled with pain relievers and is responsive to self-care.

■ **Osteoporosis.** Osteoporosis, a disease in which the bones break down and become brittle, can be a source of back pain if it results in fractures of the vertebrae. Muscles of the spine go into spasm because of these fractures. If the fractures become numerous, the spine can shorten and curve, pressing on nerves. Postmenopausal women are at the greatest risk for osteoporosis. Drug treatment is currently available to slow the

(continued on next page)

(continued)

progression of the disease, and self-care may be helpful.

■ **Pregnancy.** Though not a medical condition or illness, pregnancy can be hard on the back. Pregnancy encourages a swaybacked posture, in which the forward tilt of the lower back is exaggerated. This posture puts extra pressure on spinal discs of the lumbar (lower) region of the spine. The condition can be made worse when the mother's body produces a muscle- and ligament-relaxing hormone called relaxin for purposes of easing delivery. As a result, swayback becomes even more pronounced, irritating spinal discs even further and causing pain. Because drugs are not recommended during pregnancy, self-care is the primary form of treatment for pregnancy-related backache. Most problems disappear after delivery.

■ **Scoliosis.** Scoliosis occurs when the spine develops lateral (side-to-side) curves. The spine takes on the shape of a C if just one curve develops or an S if two curves form. It usually begins in adolescence before the vertebrae fuse, though the condition can, in rare cases, develop during adulthood. Pain can result from undue pressure that the lateral curve exerts on spinal discs. Treatment, if necessary, involves either immobilizing the spine with a brace until the bones fuse or fusing the spine surgically.

■ **Spinal stenosis.** This chronic condition, in which inflammation narrows the spinal column to the point that it encroaches on the spinal cord, sometimes develops as a result of osteoarthritis. Symptoms usually include pain and weakness in the legs and back. Spinal stenosis also can result from an abnormally narrow spinal column at birth, a bone disorder called Paget's disease, or even a herniated spinal disc. Treatment depends on the type and cause of the stenosis and may require surgery.

■ **Spondylolysis and spondylolisthesis.** These conditions result from a defect or stress fracture in one of the spine's facet joints that causes the adjoining vertebrae to move about too

(continued on next page)

(continued)

freely (spondylolysis). Over time, this excessive movement can stretch spinal muscles and ligaments to a point where the affected vertebrae slide forward (spondylolisthesis). Sometimes the "slipped" vertebrae slide far enough to press on a spinal nerve, causing pain. Treatment includes traction to align and immobilize the spine, physical therapy, and, in severe cases, surgery to fuse the affected vertebrae into their proper positions.

■ **Tumors.** Tumors, either malignant (cancerous) or benign (noncancerous), may occur in the spine, though this happens very rarely. These growths can affect virtually any part of the spine–the vertebrae, discs, ligaments, muscles, and even the synovial fluid and membranes within facet joints–and can originate in these areas or metastasize (spread) from cancers elsewhere in the body. Treatment includes surgery to remove the growth and drug or radiation treatment to eradicate cancer.

■ **Whiplash.** "Whiplash" is a term used to describe injury to the cervical (upper) section of the spine caused by rapid acceleration or deceleration, resulting usually from a car collision. Damage usually takes the form of injury to the facet joints of the vertebrae and related muscles and ligaments, but rarely is damage done to spinal discs or the vertebrae themselves. Treatment includes immobilization of the neck, use of pain relievers, and physical therapy.

spinal nerve along another part of the spinal column. Or the gelatinous center of the disc may break open, spilling its highly irritating contents and causing nerve irritation. Depending on the degree to which a disc has been damaged and the nerves affected, surgery may be required to remove all or part of the disc. But even in the most serious cases, self-care and prevention techniques can still be helpful before and after treatment.

And how can you know if your pain is due to injury to a spinal disc? As with an injury to a facet joint, a seemingly minor incident can bring it on. But unlike facet joint pain, the pain will be moderate at first and will worsen in the few days after your injury. Also in contrast to facet joint pain, your back will hurt more when you lean forward and less when you bend backward. Another distinguishing characteristic of disc injury is that even though your pain may improve substantially within about a week, it may not disappear entirely, instead lingering in a milder form for weeks or even months. Pain from sciatica, which also occurs with facet joint problems, also may be felt shooting into your buttocks and thighs. If you've injured a disc to a point where it's pressing on a spinal nerve, you may feel pain all the way into your feet and toes. Nerve involvement of this type can be serious because it can damage nerve function permanently if not relieved. Fortunately, nerve impingement of this type is fairly rare, occurring only in about 10 percent of all back pain cases, according to Hall.

The Good News About Your Bad Back

As prevalent as back pain is, it's also highly treatable and preventable. According to a 1994 review of some 3,900 studies on back pain by the U.S. Agency for Health Care Policy and Research (AHCPR), substantial relief can be achieved through self-care in 90 percent of backache cases. That's what we need to keep in mind even in our times of greatest duress.

The very fact that we're responsible for causing most of our back pain means we're also capable of curing most of it. In this book, we show you that maintaining a pain-free back can be surprisingly easy. In fact, there are only three basic steps: (1) Respond appropriately when your back goes on the fritz, (2) keep your back strong to help minimize its inherent weaknesses, and (3) learn to use your back in less damaging ways.

For those who are already suffering, Chapter 2 gets right into how to handle a backache the correct way, from the onset of the pain through recovery. For those who are between bouts of back pain or at risk for attack, Chapter 3 provides valuable prevention tips—information that's perhaps even more important because studies show that once backache does strike, it's four times more likely to strike again. You'll learn that preventing back pain is very much within your control. Plus, Chapter 4 explains new treatments and possibilities on the horizon for back-pain sufferers.

So if you do suffer from back pain, either occasionally or chronically, remember that you can take charge. To find out how, read on.

2 Treating Backache

Now that we've seen what can cause back pain, it's time to learn what to do when it strikes. How you respond to your pain—both immediately as well as in the days and weeks following your attack—can make a significant difference in how quickly and thoroughly you recover. In fact, a study published in the August 1994 issue of the *Annals of Internal Medicine* found that back patients whose physicians taught them how to care for their conditions fared better than patients whose doctors were more inclined to prescribe bed rest and medications as the mainstays of their treatment.

So find a comfortable chair—preferably one with armrests and good lower-back support—and prepare to take charge of your pain. Remember: The more you can do for yourself when back pain strikes, the faster and more complete your recovery is apt to be.

"Patients with back pain who have the best chance for recovery are those with an informed and positive attitude," writes Harris H. McIlwain, M.D., in *Winning With Back Pain.** More and more, research is beginning to show that the greater the role you play in the management of your back pain, the greater the success you'll likely have. For the vast majority of back problems, you can be your own best back doctor.

---

* New York: John Wiley and Sons, 1994.

First Things First: Immediate Steps to Ease the Pain

Rule out conditions that need medical care.

When it comes to self-care of back pain, the odds are in your favor. According to a 1994 review of some 3,900 studies on back pain by the U.S. Agency for Health Care Policy and Research (AHCPR), only 10 percent of back problems require a doctor's care rather than self-care. But before you commit yourself to self-care, read through the following guidelines on when to consult a physician—and keep these guidelines in mind throughout your recovery—just to be sure you're part of the majority who can handle care at home.

If your back pain can be characterized in any of the following ways or is being accompanied by any of the following symptoms, you should seek professional care.

■ Your back pain is constant and severe and hasn't improved after three days of bed rest.

■ Your back pain is moderate but has persisted for more than a month despite efforts to relieve it.

■ Your back pain disappears only to reappear on a regular basis.

■ Your back pain is accompanied by a noticeable change in your bowel habits.

■ In addition to your back pain, you're experiencing weakness in one or both of your legs.

■ In addition to your back pain, you're having trouble raising the toes on one or both of your feet.

■ Your back pain is accompanied by unexplainable weight loss.

■ Your back pain is accompanied by a fever that is not associated with a cold or flu.

■ Your back pain is accompanied by swelling in joints such as your fingers, wrists, elbows, ankles, or knees.

■ Your back pain has been waking you up at night.

The above symptoms could indicate nerve impingement in need of medical attention or an infection, illness, or other condition also requiring medical care. (For tips on taking your back to the doctor, see "Beyond Self-Care: Traditional and Nontraditional Intervention" later in this chapter.)

Know also that self-care is an important part of recovering from a back injury, whether or not you're being treated by a professional. If you do seek a practitioner's advice, ask how you can incorporate self-care tips into your treatment program for a fast recovery.

Stop what you're doing.

When back pain first strikes, job one is to stop whatever motion brought on the pain—"and the sooner the better," says Hamilton Hall, M.D., orthopedic surgeon and founder of the Canadian Back Institute in Toronto, in his book *The Back Doctor.** While this advice may seem to be simple common sense, too many people ignore back pain, perhaps in favor of wrapping up a tennis match or finishing up the yard work or some other activity.

You should know that the longer you continue to aggravate the source of your pain, the more your back muscles will tighten in their attempt to immobilize your injured area and the longer your recovery will take. What you want to avoid at all costs, says Hall, is a condition known as edema, whereby muscular spasms become so severe and prolonged that the affected muscles begin to retain fluid. This swells the muscles, increases their irritability, and creates even greater discomfort.

Don't panic.

Regardless of what has brought on your back pain—an afternoon working in the garden or just bending over to tie your shoe—the sooner you can stop what you're doing, the better. But it's also im-

* Toronto: McClelland and Stewart, 1987.

portant to put your mind at ease, say Alfred O. Bonati, M.D., director and chief surgeon of the Gulf Coast Orthopedic Center Institute for Special Surgery in Hudson, Florida, and Shirley Linde, Ph.D., in their book *No More Back Pain.** Becoming tense or starting to panic can cause muscles that may already be in spasm to tighten even further, Bonati and Linde say.

First of all, assure yourself that your pain will pass. According to AHCPR guidelines, 9 out of 10 people with lower-back problems recover within one month, and most recover sooner. Concurs Hall, "Without exception, every acute attack eventually subsides. What can be helpful to remember, too, is that as long as you take the right steps to look after your back following an acute episode of pain, no attack in the future will ever be as severe."

If this optimistic information doesn't bring an end to your stress, see the tips on reducing stress and using relaxation techniques in Chapter 3 for a quick way to help your stress–and your pain–subside.

Get into position.

Relax your body as well as your mind when back pain strikes–and again, the sooner the better to minimize muscular spasms. "Assume and remain in the most soothing rest position you can find," says Hall. No single position is best for all cases of back pain since no two cases are alike, so "experiment gently until you find a position that works for you," he advises.

If your pain is being caused by pressure on a spinal disc, lie on your stomach while supporting yourself with your elbows so that your back is slightly arched. If your problem is with a facet joint, sit on the floor with your knees pulled into your chest. As a third alternative, try the position that Hall himself adopts when his own back goes on one of its periodic blinks: Simply lie on the floor on your back with your feet and calves resting on the seat of a chair. Your thighs should be vertical to the floor, while your calves should be horizontal. Put a pillow beneath your head and/or buttocks for greater comfort.

Whichever of these positions works best for you, breathe deeply

---

* New York: Pharos, 1991.

and slowly and remain in the position until the most acute phase of your attack has passed, which in most cases shouldn't be more than 10 to 15 minutes. If you feel well enough following this period, try some gentle stretching exercises to further ease your pain (see tip below).

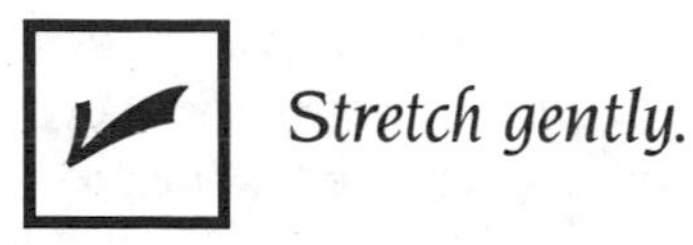

Stretch gently.

Try a session of strategic stretching, which often can stop backache in its tracks. Stretching is especially useful if the pain is due merely to stiffness from sitting in the same place for too long or to a minor muscle spasm caused by an activity you're not accustomed to doing—shoveling snow or hand waxing your kitchen floor, for example.

Here are some stretches that Bonati and Linde suggest for relieving backaches of this relatively benign nature, though they also can work to reduce the pain of more serious conditions. Do not continue these stretches, however, if it quickly becomes clear that they are making your pain worse.

■ **Standing arch.** Slowly stand up, place your palms in the small of your back just above your buttocks, and lean gently backward. Repeat five or six times or until your condition has noticeably improved.

This is perhaps the simplest maneuver for relieving most cases of backache, especially those caused by prolonged sitting or working in a stooped position.

■ **Press-up.** Lie facedown on the floor with your arms crossed underneath you. Hold this position for several minutes to help your back muscles relax. Then, as if you were about to do a push-up, place your palms on the floor, shoulder-width apart. Press slowly upward until your arms are straight, keeping your thighs in contact with the floor as you do. Hold this position for about 10 seconds, then return to your starting position for a short rest. Repeat until your condition has improved.

This is a good maneuver for relieving the pain of an acute back attack brought on by undue pressure on a spinal disc, but as with the exercise above, it also can be effective at relieving general stiffness following long periods of sitting or working in a bent-over posture.

■ **Jackknife.** While lying on your back, grasp one leg behind the knee and slowly pull it as far as you can toward your chest, keeping your back on the floor as you do. Hold this position for 10 seconds, relax, then repeat with the other leg. Repeat until your condition has improved. You may experience some mild discomfort with your first few pulls, but your pain should lessen with each one you do.

This maneuver can help relieve acute back pain caused by irritation to a facet joint of the spine, but as with the exercises above, it also can be helpful in relieving general stiffness in the lower back.

■ **Tennis ball massage.** This is a good follow-up to the stretching exercises described above. Lie down on top of two tennis balls so that they're positioned in the small of your back on either side of your spine. Then, while breathing deeply, shift your body slightly from side to side and head to toe. The tennis balls rolling beneath you will have a massaging effect on your back.

Ice your pain.

Ice the area of soreness as soon as possible after an attack of back pain has occurred to reduce pain. In addition to numbing nerves within the injured area and helping to relax tense muscles, icing reduces blood flow and, hence, the swelling and inflammation that can be additional sources of pain, says McGill University professor of psychology Ronald Melzack, Ph.D., in *The Doctors Book of Home Remedies*.* There also is a benefit once the icing is stopped, Melzack says–an increase in blood flow to the injured area that leads to accelerated healing.

Icing is best done for approximately seven to eight minutes at a time (or until a state of numbness has been reached) every few hours for a period of two days. After this 48-hour period, apply heat to aid the healing process further (see tip below).

You can make a handy icing device by freezing water in a paper cup and tearing off the cup's rim so that approximately an inch of ice is exposed, leaving the bottom of the cup as a handle. Wrap the device in a plastic bag or towel, and rub the injured area in a circular

---

* Emmaus, Pa.: Rodale, 1990.

fashion until the area is numb. If you feel a burning sensation while icing, stop for a minute or so until it subsides, then continue until numbness is achieved. Another method of icing is to apply a plastic bag of ice cubes or frozen vegetables that has been wrapped in a wet towel. Flexible, reusable cold compresses are also available in drugstores. Secure the bag or compress over the area of soreness for about 20 minutes or until numbness occurs.

End the Agony: Managing Your Pain

Turn up the heat.

While the purpose of icing is to restrict blood flow—important in the early stages of backache to limit swelling—heat has just the opposite effect: It increases blood flow and hence the delivery of oxygen and other healing nutrients to injured tissues. Heat therapy, therefore, is best begun several days—usually 48 hours after the onset of an acute attack of back pain.

"Moist heat, in the form of a hot water bottle wrapped in a wet towel, is generally considered more helpful than dry heat from a heating pad," say Glenn S. Rothfeld, M.D., and coauthor Suzanne LeVert in *Natural Medicine for Back Pain.** Rothfeld, clinical instructor at Tufts University School of Medicine and founder and medical director of Spectrum Medical Arts in Arlington, Massachusetts, and LeVert recommend applying heat two to three times a day for 15 to 30 minutes at a time.

Alternate ice and heat.

After the first two days of icing your back, you might try using ice and heat alternately, which some people report brings greater relief than either therapy alone, says Edward A. Abraham, M.D., assistant clinical

---

* Emmaus, Pa.: Rodale, 1996.

professor of orthopedics at the University of California, Irvine, in his book *Freedom From Back Pain.** These therapies work together as counter-irritants, meaning they create a lesser "pain" in order to distract the body from its greater pain. The combination of ice and heat helps to disguise back pain by stimulating, then restimulating, the nerves that would ordinarily relay pain signals to the brain. If you want to try this method, Abraham recommends a cycle of 30 minutes of ice followed by 30 minutes of heat.

Soak your soreness.

Relieve the discomfort of muscles in spasm during the acute stages of backache (as well as during chronic episodes) with a hot shower, bath, or soak in a whirlpool. Such therapy—known as hydrotherapy—increases blood flow to the injured area and has the same counter-irritating effect of applied heat, distracting the body from its own pain. In addition, hydrotherapy is a form of relaxation therapy, working to calm the mind and promote the body's natural healing mechanisms.

A shower usually is preferable to a bath in the early stages of a back attack because of the pain that can be caused by getting in and out of a tub, plus the discomfort of the sitting position that a bath requires, says Hamilton Hall, M.D., orthopedic surgeon and founder of the Canadian Back Institute in Toronto, in his book *The Back Doctor.* "Stand with your back to the shower head while propping one of your feet up on a low stool," he suggests.

If you have access to a hot tub or whirlpool large enough to allow you to stand or stretch out, by all means use it, he adds. Water naturally supports the body, taking some of the pressure off tight muscles. Positioning yourself so that the whirlpool's pulsating currents come in direct contact with your area of soreness can be especially soothing, Hall says.

---

* Emmaus, Pa.: Rodale, 1986.

Use ointments and rubs prudently.

Ointments–for example, Ben-Gay, Tiger Balm, and Icy Hot–also can help reduce the discomfort of most cases of common backache. But be forewarned that there is nothing curative about the pain relief these products achieve. Ointments work in the same way that ice and heat do–merely as counterirritants that help mask back pain by offering irritations of their own to keep the nerves busy. The ointments themselves do not penetrate deeply enough to have any true healing effect on underlying tissue.

Still, you should observe some precautions when using these products. Do not use them in conjunction with heating pads or heat lamps. Also, do not cover an area to which they've been applied with tight wraps or any fabric less breathable than normal clothing. The heat they create is very real and can cause burning if the area is not adequately ventilated.

Take the most effective over-the-counter medications.

If you're looking to the medicine cabinet for a solution to your back pain, know that experts consider the most effective over-the-counter (OTC) medications for backache to be ibuprofen (for example, Advil, Nuprin, Medipren, and Motrin IB), aspirin (for example, Bayer and Empirin), and acetaminophen (for example, Tylenol, Datril, and Panadol), in that order. This conclusion is based on a 1994 review of some 3,900 studies on back pain done by the U.S. Agency for Health Care Policy and Research.

Ibuprofen and aspirin generally are superior to acetaminophen because they're better at reducing inflammation within injured tissue, a frequent problem in back pain involving arthritis. In back pain due to muscular injury, moreover, these anti-inflammatory powers can reduce pain while aiding the healing process.

Several OTC medications on the market are specifically designed for back pain; however, experts say that there's no evidence that these products are any more effective than standard pain relievers in treating back pain. One example of such a product is Doan's pills, which contain the active ingredient magnesium salicylate.

Keep in mind that ibuprofen and aspirin can be irritating to the stomach and small intestine, so always take them with food and try not to exceed six tablets in any 24-hour period. Acetaminophen, though easier on the stomach, also has drawbacks—it can cause kidney damage if taken for long periods and liver damage if taken in conjunction with alcohol—so be careful when using this medication, as well. Side effects also can increase the longer the medications are taken, so be careful if treating a case of chronic back pain. Finally, remember that aspirin should not be taken by those under the age of 19 without a doctor's recommendation because of the risk of Reye's syndrome, a potentially fatal condition.

A general rule for taking any pain medication is simply this: Take the smallest dose possible for the shortest period of time possible—never for longer than a few weeks without seeing your doctor. This is because pain medications do nothing to correct the cause of your pain; they only mask the symptoms of your pain.

Think twice before taking your back to bed.

Resist the temptation to take your aching body to bed when backache strikes. Most experts now agree that it's not time to throw in the towel until all other, less drastic pain-relieving measures have failed. The reason for this is quite simple: In most cases of acute lower-back pain, bed rest does more harm than good.

Perhaps the most convincing proof of that surprising news comes from a carefully controlled study that was done in Finland and reported in the *New England Journal of Medicine* in February 1995. The study found that people suffering from acute lower-back pain who went about their daily routines as best they could recovered more quickly and more completely than patients with similar conditions who were assigned the seemingly more sensible treatment of two days of bed rest. In fact, the group who carefully went about their daily affairs fared better than another group of patients assigned to a special program of back exercises.

"This is not to suggest that you should remain on your feet if your pain is truly incapacitating, but it does point to drawbacks of immobilizing yourself totally," says Warren Scott, M.D., founder and chief of the Division of Sports Medicine at the Kaiser Permanente Medical Center in Santa Clara, California. But the problem with bed rest is that while it rests the muscles of the back, it also weakens them, explains Garth Russell, M.D., a professor of orthopedic surgery at the University of Missouri, in the May 1994 issue of *Muscle and Fitness* magazine. "As a general rule, for every day a patient spends in bed, it takes another day to get the muscles back to normal, so we're now encouraging patients to get moving as soon as possible," Russell says.

So unless your pain is truly unbearable, you're better off working through it than letting it land you in bed. And if you decide you do need to rest in bed, "at least get up and walk around every couple of hours or so," recommends Scott. "This can help prevent much of the muscular weakening that otherwise would occur."

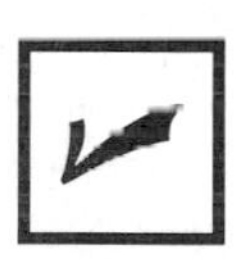

Bed down the right way.

Whether you're grabbing a quick nap, tucking in for the night, or heading for the bed because of a particularly severe attack of back pain, choose the position that will benefit you the most. The goal of bed rest is to take as much pressure off the spine as possible, so you need to adopt a position that does that best. Different conditions, of course, require different positions to accomplish this decompression, but in all things, let your comfort be your guide, says Hamilton Hall, M.D., orthopedic surgeon and founder of the Canadian Back Institute in Toronto, in his book *The Back Doctor.* If a position reduces your pain, it's reducing pressure on the components of your spine responsible for your pain.

Experiment with various positions with that in mind. If your pain is being caused by a problem with a facet joint, lying on your stomach probably will feel best, Hall says. But if your problem is with a spinal disc, lying on your back with a pillow beneath your knees or on your side curled up with a pillow between your knees probably will bring you the most relief.

Know how to get out of bed.

This can seem easy enough when your back is healthy, but it can be torture when it's not. To ease the agony of this otherwise routine maneuver, avoid sitting up and spinning your body as you normally might. Instead, pretend you're a log (which shouldn't be difficult) and roll out of bed, says Mike Hage, M.S., P.T., of the Rehabilitation Institute of Chicago, in *The Back Pain Book*.*

While lying on your back with your knees bent at a 90-degree angle, slide yourself close enough to the edge of your bed so that your knees will be hanging over the edge when you roll over. Once you do roll over, gently lower your feet to the floor as you also slowly sit up sideways, using your arms to help you.

Don't brace yourself.

Elastic braces—also called back corsets or back belts—are sometimes recommended to support the spine during the early and most painful stages of back pain and help take strain off the muscles in spasm. These braces are thought to work by compressing the abdomen, which takes some of the pressure off the spine, and they also act as reminders to take it easy.

However, some experts warn against back braces because there is no scientific evidence that proves they are effective in either treating or preventing back pain. With this lack of evidence in mind, the U.S. Agency for Health Care Policy and Research recommends against the use of back belts as a treatment, and the National Institute for Occupational Safety and Health recommends against their use to prevent injury. According to research, using a back belt may put a strain on the cardiovascular system. Research also indicates that people who wear the belts are more likely to take on heavier tasks than they can handle.

Still, some people may find relief in a back brace or corset.

---

* Atlanta: Peachtree, 1992.

What it comes down to is this: "If a back brace or corset helps your acute pain, use it but only as needed," says Harris H. McIlwain, M.D., in *Winning With Back Pain*. "Remove it when you exercise and as soon as you experience some improvement." In any case, back braces should not be used once pain has subsided. The reason? Muscles responsible for supporting the spine can grow weak if a back brace is worn too long or too often, thus making future attacks all the more likely.

The Road to Recovery: Tips for Health and Healing

Massage—there's the rub.

Treat yourself to a massage during the early stages of a backache. Massage helps loosen muscles in spasm, and it can increase blood flow to the injured area, thus facilitating healing. For optimum results, it's best to seek treatment from a licensed practitioner of massage, but a willing family member or friend also can be enlisted.

If you try massage at home, have your amateur masseur or masseuse apply rubbing alcohol or witch hazel to your back, then begin rubbing and kneading the muscles in your area of soreness using long, firm strokes. He or she "should rub toward the heart using fingertips, thumbs, knuckles, elbows—whatever feels good to you," say Alfred O. Bonati, M.D., director and chief surgeon of the Gulf Coast Orthopedic Center Institute for Special Surgery in Hudson, Florida, and Shirley Linde, Ph.D., in their book *No More Back Pain*. For a particularly pain-dispersing experience, have your masseur locate and then press into your areas of greatest tenderness for a period of 7 to 10 seconds, Bonati and Linde say. You'll experience some discomfort momentarily, but the technique often can help loosen muscles that softer strokes cannot.

For more information on massage or the names of qualified practitioners in your area, contact the American Massage Therapy Association at 820 Davis Street, Suite 100, Evanston, IL 60201-4444; 312-761-AMTA. You can also contact the National Certification Board for Therapeutic Massage and Bodywork at 8201 Greensboro Drive, Suite 300, McLean, VA 22102; 800-296-0664 or reach them on-line at http://www.ncbtmb.com.

Enjoy therapeutic sex.

If approached in the right way, sex usually does more to help than hurt those with back pain. Many arthritis patients, for example, report that they achieve "six to eight hours of relief from pain following sexual activity," say Bonati and Linde. Better yet, the thrusting motions that sex involves, if done gently, can actually help strengthen back muscles, the authors say. To enjoy such therapeutic effects, however, certain precautions should be taken. Exceptionally "acrobatic" positions should be avoided, as should any movements that are sudden or jarring or that cause the back to be greatly arched. Best for most back-pain sufferers–male and female alike–is a "spoon" position, Bonati and Linde say, with both partners lying on their sides, knees slightly bent. It also can be helpful to prepare for sex by loosening up with a hot bath or gentle massage, they say.

If pain does become a problem during sex, stop, wait for the pain to subside, and try again in a more accommodating position, Bonati and Linde suggest. But if your pain persists and is severe, discontinue your efforts and consult with your doctor.

Eat foods that help your back to heal.

Difficulty with elimination brought on by constipation can put undue pressure on even a healthy spine, so you certainly want to avoid this problem when you're recovering from an injury to your back, says Edward A. Abraham, M.D., assistant clinical professor of orthopedics at the University of California, Irvine, in his book *Freedom From Back Pain*. Hence, it is important to eat foods that are "easy to digest, process, and eliminate," he says. This means gradually adding more high-fiber foods such as fruits, vegetables, and whole-grain cereals and breads to your diet and cutting back on fried foods and high-fat proteins such as beef, pork, and cheese. Also, try to drink at least eight glasses of water a day to keep you "moving," Abraham says.

Work your way up to normal activity.

Once the worst of your back pain is over, the next challenge becomes one of getting back to normal. How fast do you go? You go as quickly but as comfortably as you can. What you want to avoid is the vicious circle of inactivity leading to muscular weakness, leading to more pain, leading to more inactivity and more weakness and more pain, and so on, say Bonati and Linde. The key to successful recovery is to work back into your normal routine gradually and cautiously, they say, doing what you can while learning to avoid what you can't do. Be especially careful of lifting, for example, and avoid becoming unduly stressed or physically fatigued. Also, be careful of long periods of sitting and any sports that may cause you pain, especially those such as tennis or golf that require excessive twisting of the spine. "Let your pain be your guide," Bonati and Linde emphasize. If an activity hurts, either stop or make adjustments in your form. Generally speaking, the best activities to pursue during the recovery phase of back pain are walking and swimming (the backstroke, especially), they say.

Once you're back on your feet, your real work has only just begun because a back once injured is more easily injured again. You will need to strengthen your back and learn proper body mechanics to prevent attacks from occurring in the future.

Beyond Self-Care: Traditional and Nontraditional Intervention

See your family doctor first.

As we've said before, professional care for back pain is usually not necessary. However, there are some cases in which it would be best to seek treatment from a physician or other health-care practitioner.

If you're considering seeing a professional, you can use the guidelines discussed in "First Things First: Immediate Steps to Ease the Pain" at the beginning of this chapter to help evaluate your case.

Start with your family doctor when seeking the best treatment for your backache. After all, he or she is best informed of your medical history–one of the most important keys to deciphering the cause of your back pain. If you do not have a family doctor, check with your local hospital or medical society for a reputable practitioner or back-pain clinic in your area. If you belong to a managed-care plan, you'll need to see a practitioner who belongs to the plan for treatment or a referral.

After taking your medical history, your practitioner will perform a physical examination. In most cases, you'll be asked to do some simple exercises such as walking across the room, reaching for your toes, and touching your finger to the tip of your nose. Your reflexes and muscle strength will be checked, and the doctor may press an area on your leg or foot to see if you can feel the pressure. You may also be asked to lie down and raise your leg, keeping it straight, or to straighten your leg while sitting on the examining table to see if your sciatic nerve is affected. These tests, recommended by the U.S. Agency for Health Care Policy and Research (AHCPR), are designed to rule out any serious medical conditions and help diagnose the problem.

In most cases, a primary-care practitioner will provide self-care information and possibly a prescription for medication or another type of therapy. Your family doctor is also in the best position to recommend other forms of therapy if it becomes clear that your problem is not within his or her scope of practice.

Weigh your diagnostic options.

While a medical history and physical examination are the starting points for medically treating back pain, there are other methods available to help you and your practitioner discover the source of your back pain. If you've been suffering from back pain for more than one month, talk to your doctor about which of the following tests might be right–or wrong–for you.

■ **Bone scan.** In this procedure, a radioactive substance that adheres to the bone is injected into the body. Then an imaging device is used to create pictures of the highlighted bones. Bone scans are used to diagnose fractures, infections, abnormal bone growth of the spine, and degeneration of the vertebrae.

■ **CT (computerized tomography) and MRI (magnetic resonance imaging) scans.** A CT scan uses x-rays (see below) to create a three-dimensional image of the back and spine, while an MRI uses magnetic fields to create cross-sectional images. These techniques are generally used only for diagnosis when symptoms are severe enough to consider surgery. (See "The Last Resort: Surgery" at the end of this chapter.)

■ **Discography.** This is an invasive test that involves the injection of a dye into a spinal disc to diagnose an abnormal or deteriorating disc. According to the AHCPR, this test is usually not necessary because the same information often can be obtained using a noninvasive CT or MRI scan.

■ **Electrophysiologic tests.** These tests involve the use of electrodes to monitor the electrical activity of a muscle; the information is then used to assess nerve function. This can be done by inserting a needle into a muscle or by attaching the electrode to the surface of the skin.

■ **Thermography.** This noninvasive test creates images of the body using temperature differences. The AHCPR reports that it is generally not considered to be an effective test for diagnosing the causes of back pain.

■ **X-ray.** An x-ray uses a low dose of radioactivity to create an image of the spine. It is used to diagnose any structural abnormalities that may be causing back pain.

Avoid prescription drugs.

Don't stray from ibuprofen, aspirin, and acetaminophen as pain relievers unless your physician gives you a good reason. There are a number of prescription drugs that practitioners commonly prescribe–

often out of habit—to relieve the symptoms of back pain. Yet according to the AHCPR's clinical guidelines, none of the commonly used prescription drugs is more effective at relieving pain than ibuprofen, aspirin, or acetaminophen (in that order)—even though prescription

SOME WELL-KNOWN DRUGS

Here is a list of prescription medications commonly prescribed for back pain, along with their possible side effects.

■ **Antidepressants.** These drugs, which include imipramine and trazodone, are prescribed for those with and without depression to treat nerve-associated pain, insomnia, and depression (often a symptom of chronic pain) related to backache. Side effects include dry mouth, drowsiness, constipation, and urinary retention.

■ **Colchicine.** This drug is used to treat back pain associated with gout, a form of arthritis brought on by high levels of uric acid in the body. Side effects include nausea, vomiting, and skin problems.

■ **Muscle relaxants.** These relatively inexpensive drugs include benzodiazepines (for example, Librium, Valium, and Xanax) and sedative medications. Side effects include drowsiness and dizziness.

■ **Opioid analgesics.** These drugs, which include acetaminophen with codeine (for example, Tylenol with codeine), have a number of side effects such as dizziness, impaired vision, fatigue, drowsiness, nausea, constipation, and inability to concentrate. In addition, they do carry a risk of physical dependence, even if taken for a short period.

■ **Oral steroids (corticosteroids).** These drugs are intended to reduce inflammation that may be triggering back pain. If used in low doses for a short period of time, corticosteroids have minimal side effects. However, long-term use or high dosage may lead to suppression of hormonal functions, hyperglycemia (high blood sugar), breakdown of bone, and suppression of the immune system.

drugs tend to cost more and have more side effects.

If a prescription drug is recommended by your doctor, be sure to find out why he or she feels you need it. Ask what the medication is intended to do and find out about possible side effects. You may even want to get a second opinion from another practitioner.

Another reason to be wary is that some of these drugs may be addictive, especially if taken for long periods of time–which is a possibility if you're dealing with chronic or recurrent back pain. If you do find yourself taking a prescription medication for good reason, be extremely careful, keeping its drawbacks in mind. Never exceed dosages of these drugs for longer periods than have been recommended by your doctor. And be sure to report any side effects that occur.

Know which back practitioners do what, and why.

If your family doctor decides that it would be in your best interest to seek treatment beyond what he or she can provide, make the most informed decision you can regarding what type of practitioner to see. This can indeed be daunting because no fewer than two dozen different types of back practitioners currently exist.

What follows is a list of those most commonly consulted, along with brief explanations of the types of treatment they offer. Keep in mind that medical practitioners may tend to stick to medical treatment such as drugs and surgery, though they may also rely on nonmedical treatments (see tip below). This might also be the time to ask your insurance company about coverage–some referrals and therapies might not be paid for under your plan.

■ **Allopathic physician (M.D.).** An allopathic physician is also known as a doctor of medicine, or an M.D.–the most mainstream sort of medical doctor. Many people will see an M.D. for an initial diagnosis, if not for follow-up treatment. M.D.'s are best equipped to diagnose the cause of your condition, particularly in cases where disease, neurological impairment, or a serious structural abnormality may be involved.

■ **Osteopathic physician (D.O.).** An osteopath is very similar to an allopathic physician, the only major difference being a matter of philosophy. Osteopathic training focuses on treating the body as a whole, concentrating on the body's joints, muscles, bones, ligaments, and tendons. Osteopaths are medical doctors, with the degree of doctor of osteopathy, who can prescribe drugs and even perform surgery, but generally they focus on treating back problems in more physical ways such as with massage and spinal manipulation.

■ **Orthopedic surgeon (orthopedist).** This is a medical doctor who's been specially trained in diagnosing and treating injuries and diseases of the bones and muscles as well as the ligaments, tendons, and joints. In addition to being trained to perform surgery when necessary, orthopedists also are versed in prescribing drugs for back pain as well as in overseeing other, more conservative treatment options.

■ **Neurosurgeon.** This is a medical doctor who specializes in surgery involving the nervous system. Neurosurgeons also are trained to prescribe drugs, but they rarely involve themselves with other forms of therapy.

■ **Neurologist.** A neurologist is a medical doctor who specializes in diagnosing problems with the nerves of the spine more so than its muscles and bones. Neurologists do not perform surgery but rely instead on other, noninvasive therapies.

■ **Physiatrist.** A physiatrist is a medical doctor who is trained in the best ways of employing nonsurgical techniques such as physical therapy, ultrasound, and deep tissue massage to treat back pain. Physiatrists frequently work in conjunction with physical therapists (see below) in implementing these treatments—and with encouraging success: Of all types of back practitioners studied in a survey of 492 back-pain sufferers conducted by writers Arthur C. Klein and Dava Sobel and reported in their book *Backache Relief*, physiatrists were found to achieve the greatest success in treating backache.* "This exceptional healer is your best bet among all practitioners—medical and nonmedical alike—for both acute and chronic back problems," Klein and Sobel report.

■ **Physical therapist.** A physical therapist is not a medical doctor but often works along with such doctors to supplement medical care. In most states, treatment by a physical therapist requires refer-

* New York: Times Books, 1985.

ral from a medical doctor, but it's a referral well made in most cases, according to the Klein and Sobel survey. "Physical therapists are by far the most successful nonmedical practitioners for helping patients with nearly any kind of back ailment," they report. Physical therapists employ a gamut of modalities including not just exercise but also relaxation techniques, postural instruction, advice on conducting daily activities, ultrasound, electrotherapy, massage, and even acupuncture in some cases. In other words, they treat not just your back but also your entire lifestyle, with varying degrees of success in approximately 75 percent of cases, Klein and Sobel report.

■ **Rheumatologist.** A rheumatologist is a medical doctor who specializes in treating the more than 100 forms of arthritis currently known to exist. Rheumatologists frequently prescribe exercise and other forms of conservative treatment, but they also have the training to prescribe drugs when conditions dictate it.

■ **Sports medicine specialist.** Practicing a relatively new medical specialty, the sports medicine specialist concentrates on treating injuries to muscles, bones, and joints primarily through rehabilitative exercise and other conservative modalities such as hydrotherapy, electrotherapy, and massage.

■ **Chiropractor (D.C.).** A chiropractor is not a medical doctor but rather a therapist with the degree of doctor of chiropractic who has been trained in spinal manipulation (see tip below). A chiropractor may be of the "straight school," meaning he or she relies on spinal manipulation alone as a therapy, or of the "mixed school," meaning spinal adjustments may be supplemented with other forms of treatment such as electrotherapy, massage, and even acupuncture.

Assess your treatment options.

Some 90 percent of back-pain sufferers in the Klein and Sobel survey started out by seeing a medical practitioner for treatment, but only about 40 percent concluded their care under one. The majority of back-pain sufferers switch to nonmedical therapies for relief, the most popular of which are briefly described below. Again, check with your insurance company to find out about your coverage before accepting treatment—many of these therapies are far from the mainstream and may not be paid for.

■ **Chiropractic therapy and spinal manipulation.** Chiropractic therapy, which employs spinal manipulation, has been found to be useful in treating back pain not associated with nerve damage and is most effective in those with acute rather than chronic back pain. In manipulation, the practitioner applies pressure on the spine in a specific way to restore the alignment and mobility of the vertebrae. The adjustment results in a popping or cracking sound, the same sound that comes with cracking the knuckles. (But remember: The sound doesn't indicate whether the correct adjustment has been made.)

Chiropractic therapy is most successful in providing short-term relief for relatively minor cases of backache (those due to muscular injury, irritation within a facet joint, or pressure on a spinal disc). It should not be enlisted to treat pain being caused by direct pressure on a spinal nerve such as in the case of a disc that has ruptured, authorities agree. Back pain of this type characteristically will be experienced as an intense burning sensation running down the side of either or both legs—a condition that spinal manipulation may actually make worse, says Warren Scott, M.D., founder and chief of the Division of Sports Medicine at the Kaiser Permanente Medical Center in Santa Clara, California.

Chiropractic therapy should not be used for back conditions involving osteoporosis, arthritis, fractures, tumors, and infections or malignancies of the spine, so "it's important to have your condition properly defined before any manipulation is attempted," says Hamilton Hall, M.D., orthopedic surgeon and founder of the Canadian Back Institute in Toronto, in his book *The Back Doctor.*

These particular conditions notwithstanding, recent studies support the effectiveness of chiropractic therapy for the treatment of lower-back pain in its most common forms. Based on a 1994 review of some 3,900 studies by the U.S. Agency for Health Care Policy and Research, chiropractic therapy was found "likely to provide symptomatic relief" if performed within a month of back-pain onset. Experts recommend seeking a different form of treatment if there is no improvement of back pain with spinal manipulation within four weeks. For more information on this therapy or a referral to a chiropractor in your area, contact the International Chiropractors Association, 1110

relief, your practitioner—and maybe you, too—might be looking toward surgery as a solution.

Even with recent advances that have been made in back surgery, back surgeons themselves say the surgical procedures should be reserved as a last resort. "The need for lumbar spine surgery is limited to 1 to 2 percent of patients in whom conservative management has failed," says David Borenstein, M.D., of the George Washington University Medical Center, in *Back Pain: Questions You Have . . . Answers You Need.** Going a step further, "half of all back surgeries performed in the United States are unnecessary," says Stephen Hochschuler, M.D., orthopedic surgeon and cofounder of the Texas Back Institute in Plano, Texas, in his book *Back in Shape.*†

This is not to say that certain conditions do not warrant and in fact demand surgical intervention, however. Most practitioners agree that surgery is required when a specific cause of back pain has been unmistakably identified as remediable by surgery, when there is significant and unrelenting pain, and when the patient has failed to respond to at least four to six weeks of nonsurgical treatment.

But even if your case fits these criteria, it is always smart to get a second opinion before consenting to surgery.

Find the best surgeon you can.

If it's decided that surgery is your best course, your next step is to make sure you're getting the best surgeon you can to perform it. Check first with your family doctor for any recommendations he or she may have. If that leaves you feeling less than confident, check with any friends you may have in the health-care industry who may have an inside word. Or try a doctor referral service in your area, or call your local hospital to find out if it has a referral service.

Beyond that, additional assurance of your surgeon's competence can and should be gauged by asking the office staff the following questions, say Richard Fraser, M.D., professor of neurosurgery

* Allentown, Pa.: People's Medical Society, 1995.
† Boston: Houghton Mifflin, 1991.

at Cornell University Medical College, and Ann Forer in their book *The Well-Informed Patient's Guide to Back Surgery*.*

■ How many of these operations has my prospective surgeon performed, and with what degree of success?

■ Will microsurgery (a less invasive form of surgery performed through a microscope) be used? What are the advantages and disadvantages of microsurgery?

■ To what degree will a resident doctor be participating in my operation?

■ What sort of outcomes may I realistically expect?

■ What sort of complications could possibly occur?

■ How can I expect to feel after the surgery, and for how long?

■ How soon can I expect to return to work?

■ What will the surgery cost?

If for any reason you feel uncomfortable with the answers you get to these questions, seek a second opinion. (In some cases, your insurance company may even require one.) A second opinion can confirm or eliminate any doubts you may have.

---

* New York: Dell, 1992.

3 Preventing Backache

In Chapter 1, we mentioned the three basic steps to maintaining a pain-free back: responding appropriately to back pain, keeping your back strong, and learning to use your back wisely. We've already seen in Chapter 2 how best to handle back pain when it strikes. Now it's time to learn how strengthening your back and keeping its best interests in mind can keep this all-too-common ailment from recurring.

Most experts agree that the key to conquering back pain lies in prevention. "Research has shown that once you have a back injury, you are four times as likely to have a recurrence," says Stephen Hochschuler, M.D., orthopedic surgeon and cofounder of the Texas Back Institute in Plano, Texas, in his book *Back in Shape*.* "The best way to treat back pain, therefore, is not after it happens, but before."

Prevention might seem like wishful thinking, given how common back pain is and how it can be brought on by activities as routine as taking out the trash. But we shouldn't be misled by this seeming "normalcy" of back pain, says Warren Scott, M.D., founder and chief of the Division of Sports Medicine at the Kaiser Permanente Medical Center in Santa Clara, California. "Yes, 80 percent of us suffer from backache, but most of these backaches could be prevented," Scott says. "Back pain is so common only because the ways we ask for it are so common. . . . Those backaches that seem to come out of nowhere actually are the result of months or even years of lesser offenses and

* Boston: Houghton Mifflin, 1991.

neglect. Our backs can take only so much before they finally cry out for help."

But by keeping our backs strong through regular exercise and learning to use our backs in the right ways, the chances of injury are greatly reduced. "Many of our back problems develop simply because we let our backs get out of condition," Hochschuler says.

So here's how to keep your back safe and in shape. If you suffer from back pain, these preventive strategies can greatly reduce your chances of suffering from more attacks in the future. As Harris H. McIlwain, M.D., author of *Winning With Back Pain*, says, preventive strategies against back pain can be of significant help even in the most extreme and chronic cases.* What makes the difference in such instances, he says, is perseverance—"the most powerful weapon against back pain of all."

Back Into Shape: Exercises for a Fit Back

Psych yourself.

Stay motivated in your back-pain prevention program, and understand how best to help your back by knowing exactly how exercise minimizes the risk of back pain. "Unlike mechanical components that wear down through the friction of repetitive movement, the body needs motion to retain motion," explains Hochschuler. Spinal discs, for example, benefit from the increased blood flow associated with exercise, and facet joints are treated to increased lubrication due to greater outputs of synovial fluid. Muscles and ligaments also are kept more limber. "Simply put, exercise is like WD-40 for the spine," Hochschuler says. "It lubricates the joints of the back as it stretches its muscles so they become less prone to being strained or torn."

But exercise does more than just stretch the muscles of the back—it strengthens them, helping to protect the facet joints and discs of the spine that rely on these muscles for protective support. There's also evidence that exercise can help strengthen the bones of

---

* New York: John Wiley and Sons, 1994.

the spine, helping to prevent osteoporosis-related fractures that can cause back pain. A study published in the December 28, 1994, issue of the *Journal of the American Medical Association* found that strength-building exercises prevented a loss of bone density in postmenopausal women while increasing balance, muscle mass, and strength.

There are also distinct benefits to exercise that strengthens the other muscles of the body—those of the abdomen, buttocks, legs, and trunk, especially. Strengthening these muscles reduces strain on the back indirectly, as their greater strength makes them more capable of sharing in the back's workload. Exercise that strengthens major muscle groups also increases endurance, thus allowing more work to be done before back muscles become fatigued, says Scott. Exercise is also a stress reliever, and as you'll find out later in this chapter, stress can cause muscle tension that increases the risk for back pain.

Stretch to increase flexibility.

Just as muscles should be strong to prevent back pain, they also should be flexible, say David Imrie, M.D., a physician specializing in occupational medicine, and Lu Barbuto, D.C., in their book *The Back Power Program.** This gives muscles (and their attendant ligaments) the ability to stretch rather than tear when stressed by activities such as bending and lifting. It also provides for greater mobility, which generally translates to less pain within the joints of the spine. Stretch daily for greater flexibility and also be sure to stretch right before you begin exercise to warm up your muscles and help prevent muscular backache. Imrie and Barbuto recommend the following exercises, to be done on a daily basis.

■ **Sling stretch.** While lying on your back, use your arms to gently pull one of your knees into your chest while your other leg remains straight. Hold this position for about 10 seconds while breathing slowly and deeply. Return your leg to the floor and repeat five times before repeating the sequence with your other leg.

■ **Side stretch.** While standing with your feet about 18 inches apart and your hands on your head, bend slowly sideways as far as

* New York: John Wiley and Sons, 1990.

you comfortably can. Hold this position as you breathe in deeply, then exhale. Straighten up when you've finished exhaling, then bend to the other side, using the same pattern of breathing. Repeat the sequence three to five times.

■ **Mad cat.** While down on your hands and knees on the floor, arch your back upward in the shape of a dome. Hold this position for a few seconds, then let your back return to a level position. Finally, arch your back downward (in a position opposite of the dome), hold for a few seconds, and return to your level position. Repeat the sequence three to five times.

Exercise your entire body.

Exercise should be balanced in the sense that all parts of the body should be strengthened equally, say Alfred O. Bonati, M.D., director and chief surgeon of the Gulf Coast Orthopedic Center Institute for Special Surgery in Hudson, Florida, and Shirley Linde, Ph.D., in their book *No More Back Pain.** Otherwise, muscular imbalances may result, preventing the body from working in the integrated manner in which it was designed, and thus leading to a risk of back pain. Their recommendation, therefore, is a two-pronged attack: 20 to 30 minutes of an aerobic activity (sustained exercise such as walking, cycling, jogging, or swimming that increases cardiovascular health) done at least three days a week for overall fitness and weight control, coupled with strength-building exercises.

The following exercises are for strengthening the muscles of the back as well as those of the abdomen, hips, and legs, which also are important in the prevention of back pain. Do these exercises at least every other day (daily would be even better), preferably after you have warmed up with your aerobic workout or done several minutes of light stretching to loosen any tight muscles. The exercises come recommended by Bonati and Linde as well as the American Academy of Orthopaedic Surgeons and other back experts.

■ **Wall slide (for strengthening the muscles of the back, hips, and legs).** Standing with your back against a wall, feet shoulder-

* New York: Pharos, 1991.

width apart, slide down into a crouch until your knees are bent at a 90-degree angle. Hold this position for five seconds, then press back up until your legs are straight. Repeat five times.

■ **Partial sit-up (for strengthening the muscles of the abdomen).** While lying on your back with your knees bent and feet flat on the floor, slowly raise your head and shoulders as you reach with your hands toward your knees. Hold this position for a few seconds, then return to your starting position. Repeat four times.

■ **Leg raise (for strengthening the muscles of the abdomen and hips).** While lying on your back with your arms at your sides, lift one leg about a foot off the floor, keeping it as straight as you can, and hold this position for a count of 10. Lower your leg to the floor, then repeat with your other leg. Repeat the sequence four times.

■ **Reverse leg raise (for strengthening the muscles of the back and hips).** This is a variation of the exercise described above. While lying on your stomach with your arms stretched above your head, raise one leg about a foot off the floor, again keeping it as straight as you can, and hold this position for a count of 10. Lower your leg to the floor, then repeat with your other leg. Repeat the sequence four times.

■ **Leg swing (for strengthening the muscles of the back and hips).** This exercise strengthens the same muscles as the exercise above but does not require that you lie on the floor. Standing behind a chair with your hands on the top of the chair back, lift your leg back and up as high as you comfortably can, keeping it as straight as you can, and hold this position for about a second. Lower your leg slowly to the floor, then repeat with your other leg. Repeat the sequence four times.

Don't bite off more than you can chew.

If exercise is such an effective deterrent, why does it sometimes bring on back pain? Because too often we overdo it, making the jump from a sedentary lifestyle to an active one, with little in between. Hochschuler, in his book *Back in Shape*, cites the example of the person who works behind a desk all week, only to leap headfirst into some sporting activity or demanding household chore on the weekend.

Such overexertion can result in back pain directly or can lay the groundwork for back pain later—as in the case of the weekend tennis zealot who gets socked with a back attack days later when picking up a small box of computer paper. Backaches that come as the result of a "final straw" incident constitute an estimated 60 percent of all backaches suffered, Hochschuler says.

The solution? Estimate your level of fitness before getting too active too quickly. If you're not following a regular fitness plan and are usually sedentary, think twice before joining in the touch football game at the family picnic or shoveling the snow from your entire sidewalk in one go. Start working toward physical fitness, as well. In his book *What to Do When It Hurts*, British sports medicine expert and former Olympian Malcolm Read, M.D., estimates that to get back into shape, most people need one month of regular physical activity for each year that they've been sedentary.*

In addition, you need to be active on a regular basis, not a sporadic one. "Our backs have to be conditioned for the activities we throw at them," Hochschuler says, and this applies to our activities of daily living as well as our weekend exploits. A back that has been strengthened through regular exercise is going to be more resilient to the everyday stresses of sitting, lifting, and standing just as it is to the rigors of a sport or weekend chore.

Don't aim for pain.

When it comes to the intensity you should employ in your exercise efforts, forget that the credo "No pain, no gain" was ever uttered, today's back experts agree. Pain of any type in any activity you do should serve as a warning sign, not a goal.

This isn't to say you shouldn't expect to experience minor discomfort from time to time, especially in the beginning stages of exercise as your body is getting warmed up. But pain of a persistent nature should be taken as a signal that your activity may be doing you more harm than good—increasing your risk for a backache. If pain

---

* Allentown, Pa.: People's Medical Society, 1997.

occurs, stop what you're doing and wait for the pain to recede. If it disappears within a few seconds, it's probably safe to continue, working through the discomfort, as long as the pain doesn't increase. However, if pain lingers for several minutes after you've stopped, take a rest or switch activities. If jogging or walking causes you pain, for example, try a non-weight-bearing activity such as cycling or swimming.

Don't be too hard on yourself.

Use comfort as your goal in your recreational and sporting activities, too, the experts say. This isn't to suggest you should restrict yourself to computer games or needlework in your leisure time, but it does mean you should be aware of which physical activities tend to be less back-friendly than others.

"Avoid sports that involve rough physical contact, or those in which there is twisting or severe arching of the back, or those where there is danger of sudden impact or jarring," Bonati and Linde say. As examples of such high-risk activities, they cite football, gymnastics, handball, horseback riding, volleyball, snowmobiling, wrestling, bowling, basketball, ice hockey, and soccer.

Also, watch out for tennis, golf, baseball, softball, and similar sports: These involve twisting motions that can stress the spine. Be sure you're adequately warmed up before engaging in these activities, and in the cases of tennis and golf, take lessons to learn proper form.

Generally, the activities that are kindest to the back are swimming and walking, Bonati and Linde say. Cycling also can be good, but the hunched-over, racing position should be avoided. Better to choose a bike with a well-padded seat and handlebars positioned to allow you to ride upright, they say.

As for jogging, one of the most jarring activities, let your comfort be your guide. Some people experience no trouble at all, while others nearly die with every stride, the authors say. You can minimize the dangers of jogging by taking these precautions: Wear high-quality, well-padded shoes; run on soft surfaces such as grass, dirt, or cinder or synthetic track; avoid downhill running; and do your best to run in an upright rather than forward-leaning posture.

Here are some other tips Bonati and Linde offer for being kinder to your back no matter which sport you pursue.

- Get your doctor's approval before starting.
- Take time to build endurance for your sport gradually.
- Try to avoid any movements that are sudden or jarring.
- Choose a sport that releases tension rather than a highly competitive sport that may be a tension producer.

Better Your Body: Personal Modifications for Back Health

Keep your weight down.

"For every pound of extra weight you have on your abdomen, it's been estimated that you put an extra five pounds of pressure on your back," Bonati and Linde report. "This means that carrying 10 extra pounds of weight up front can cause more strain on the lower back than carrying around a bowling ball all day long."

Why should excess weight in the abdominal area be so hard on the spine? Because it shifts the body's center of gravity forward, forcing the back muscles to work that much harder to keep the spine erect. This puts continual stress not just on the muscles of the back but on the spine's facet joints and discs as well.

To control your weight, avoid foods high in fat, limit your intake of "empty" calories such as those in junk foods and alcohol, and stay active. Exercise not only burns calories as you're doing it but also helps speed your body's metabolism even at rest so that you can be a better calorie burner 24 hours a day.

Give your body the support it needs.

Large breasts can increase the risk for back pain in the same way a potbelly can: Back muscles must remain chronically stressed to offset the shift in your center of gravity. In addition, the round-shouldered posture women sometimes self-consciously adopt can compound the problem, putting additional strain on the back. To prevent problems, maintain a good, upright posture and wear a brassiere with good support. For especially extreme cases, breast reduction surgery can be an effective option (approximately 40,000 of these procedures are done annually, according to the American Society of Plastic and Reconstructive Surgeons).

Check your posture—and fix it.

Bad posture can precipitate back pain by putting undue stress on the spine on a continual basis. Here are two quick tests you can do to determine if your posture needs work.

■ Stand with your back against a wall so that your heels are two inches from the wall and your shoulders and head are touching the wall. If the resulting space between the wall and the small of your back is greater than the thickness of your hand, you suffer from what's called swayback, a condition that puts unnatural stress on the facet joints at the rear of the spine.

■ Stand facing a wall so that your toes are just touching it. Keeping your normal posture, slowly lean toward the wall, noticing which part of your body makes contact first. If it's your chest, your posture is probably OK. But if it's your stomach, your posture—and probably your weight—need work.

If these tests indicate that your posture is poor, do not despair: You can improve your posture simply by paying more attention to it. All day, in everything you do, try to stand straight and tall with your head directly over your shoulders, not thrust forward. Keep your shoulder blades back, your stomach tucked in, and your pelvis tilted slightly backward to prevent swayback, which can aggravate spinal discs and facet joints. Aim for equal distribution of weight, aligning your well-postured body directly over your feet. Your feet should be parallel, exactly below the hip joints, with the toes straight ahead and the heels straight back.

Correct foot problems before they become back problems.

Foot problems can lead to back pain by making it difficult for you to stand normally or walk with a natural gait. See a podiatrist (a doctor who specializes in problems of the foot) for treatment if you suffer from bunions, ingrown toenails, corns, painful blisters or calluses, or fallen arches (flat feet), especially if the problem is affecting the way you walk.

Check your shoes, as well. Shoe problems can deprive your back of a stable foundation, possibly leading to back pain. Worst of all are shoes with exceptionally high heels because they tend to encourage swayback by pitching the body forward. Shoes that are old and worn also can be hard on the back, especially if their heels are worn unevenly on their inside or outside edges, thus pitching the spine from side to side with every step. Best for the back are shoes with low heels and cushioned soles to protect the spine by absorbing shock.

Get your vitamins.

Be sure to eat your fruits and vegetables. Aside from eating a healthy, low-fat diet for purposes of maintaining normal weight, you should take in adequate amounts of calcium, vitamin D, and vitamin C, as some research indicates this may help prevent back problems. Calcium and vitamin D are important for maintaining strong bones (such as vertebrae), and vitamin C has been shown to help in the formation of collagen, a key component of bones as well as ligaments and tendons. Good sources of calcium are dairy products (preferably low-fat or nonfat), broccoli, beans, dried peas, and fish such as sardines, in which the bones are also consumed. The best way to get vitamin D is from low-fat or nonfat milk that has been fortified with the vitamin. Good sources of vitamin C are citrus fruits, dark green leafy vegetables, tomatoes, green peppers, broccoli, cantaloupe, and strawberries.

If you have any doubts that you're getting enough calcium, vitamin D, and vitamin C naturally in your diet, supplementation would be a good idea. For most adults, the daily Recommended Dietary

Allowances for calcium, vitamin D, and vitamin C are 800 milligrams, 5 micrograms, and 60 milligrams, respectively.

If you smoke, stop.

According to a recent study done at the Medical College of Wisconsin by Howard An, M.D., smoking a pack or more of cigarettes a day tripled people's risk of suffering from disc problems in the lower back and quadrupled their risk of suffering from pain due to disc problems in the neck.

"There is pretty good evidence that nicotine interferes with blood flow to the vertebral body and around the discs," says Augustus A. White III, M.D., professor of orthopedic surgery at Harvard Medical School, in his book *Your Aching Back*.* This may cause abnormalities in the normal functioning of the discs, with back pain being the result. Add the chronic pressure on spinal discs caused by the inordinate amount of coughing that smokers do, and the link between smoking and back pain becomes clearer yet, says White. The good news is that when people stop smoking, the risk of back trouble returns to normal within five years.

Quitting smoking is difficult but well worth it—especially when the risks of lung disease, cancer, and a number of other conditions are added to the risk of backache caused by smoking. For more information on how to quit, contact the American Lung Association, 1740 Broadway, New York, NY 10019; 800-586-4872.

Boardroom to Bedroom: Tips for at Work and at Home

Sit less.

Sitting, as we saw in Chapter 1, puts 50 percent more pressure on spinal discs as standing. Done in a slouching fashion or in a chair that

---

* New York: Simon and Schuster, 1990.

provides inadequate support, it can be even harder on the back than lifting. Over time, pressure causes spinal discs to bulge, increasing the risk of impingement on a spinal nerve. Eventually, the disc may herniate, or rupture, from the accumulation of pressure.

Obviously, you can't and shouldn't avoid sitting altogether, but you should avoid sitting for extended periods of time. If your job requires you to sit, "make it a priority to get up from your desk or workstation at least once every 30 minutes to take a short break lasting a minute or two," recommends Robert K. Cooper, Ph.D., in his book *The Performance Edge*.* Even if all you can manage is to stand up and walk around a bit, you'll be increasing circulation as well as decreasing pressure on spinal discs.

If getting up is inappropriate or impossible, lean forward periodically, and if possible, lower your head to your knees for a few minutes, suggest Bonati and Linde in *No More Back Pain*.

Standing too much can be hard on your back, too. If your job demands that you stand for extended periods, lessen the strain on your back by keeping one foot slightly raised (about six inches high) on a small stool, say Richard Fraser, M.D., professor of neurosurgery at Cornell University Medical College, and Ann Forer in their book *The Well-Informed Patient's Guide to Back Surgery*.† "Also alternate your feet from time to time, and try to walk around for at least a few steps as often as possible," they say.

Sit better.

As hard on the back as sitting can be, however, it can be made easier if it's done using a position that maintains the natural curve of the spine, says Edward A. Abraham, M.D., assistant clinical professor of orthopedics at the University of California, Irvine, in his book *Freedom From Back Pain*.‡ To achieve this position, place a small cylindrical pillow or rolled-up towel between the chair and the small of your back (the lumbar region) so that the only parts of your body in actual contact with the back of the chair are your upper back and buttocks.

---

* Boston: Houghton Mifflin, 1991.
† New York: Dell, 1992.
‡ Emmaus, Pa.: Rodale, 1986.

Also, keep your head and neck held erect and keep your feet flat on the floor or, better yet, on a low stool or several phone books so that they are slightly raised. This puts your knees slightly higher than your hips, a position that lends to the natural curve of the spine. Don't sit with one ankle resting on the opposite thigh, recommends the September 1994 issue of *Men's Health*. This shortens leg muscles, curves the spine, and pinches the nerves in the leg, which may lead to back pain.

When getting up out of a chair, try to use your arms as much as possible to reduce pressure on your spine, says Mike Hage, M.S., P.T., of the Rehabilitation Institute of Chicago, in *The Back Pain Book*.* If your chair has armrests, use them to press yourself into an upright position. If there are no armrests, press up from the seat of the chair.

Know a good chair when you see one.

How long you sit and how you sit can make a substantial difference in your risk for back pain, so it's no surprise that where you sit also matters.

First, avoid chairs that abuse the back. Worst of all are chairs that provide little or no support for the lumbar (lower) part of the spine—softly cushioned, low-slung lounge chairs and couches, or seats with no backs at all such as stadium bleachers and piano benches. Lumbar support is important for helping the muscles of the back in their job of maintaining the back's natural lumbar curve. Without this support, the back's muscles can become painfully fatigued. Worse yet, the slouching position that often comes with such fatigue allows the spine's discs to become unduly compressed, leading to additional pain.

You can solve the problem of no lumbar support in the case of backless benches by using a device known aptly as a stadium chair, which has a seat and a back but no legs. In the case of a painfully soft couch, however, you may have do the best you can to improve its support by propping whatever cushions may be available behind your lower back. Otherwise, it may be best to "just say no" and sit cross-legged on the floor, instead.

---

* Atlanta: Peachtree, 1992.

Second, seek the most perfect chair possible. There are certain basic features to look for in a chair that can substantially reduce the hazards of sitting. In a desk chair, look for adjustability in height so that you can sit with your knees slightly higher than your hips, the position that helps maintain the spine's natural lumbar curve. The chair also should provide good lumbar support for your spine and have armrests set at a comfortable height. The chair's seat should be padded yet firm enough (and wide enough) to allow you to shift positions easily, and it should be deep enough to support about three-quarters of your thighs.

As for the best "easy chair" for your back, look again for firmness, good lumbar support, comfortable armrests, and a seat shallow enough to allow your feet to reach the floor. In a survey of 492 back-pain sufferers done by writers Arthur C. Klein and Dava Sobel and reported in their book *Backache Relief*, respondents generally preferred easy chairs that could be adjusted to allow them to sit with their knees higher than their hips.*

Chairs on which you kneel rather than sit have been advertised as good for back-pain sufferers—and they can be, because the kneeling position helps sustain the spine's natural lumbar curve, says Hamilton Hall, M.D., orthopedic surgeon and founder of the Canadian Back Institute in Toronto, in his book *The Back Doctor*.† Hall cautions, however, that these chairs can put a substantial load on the knees if used for extended periods. "Like many devices designed to help the back," says Hall, "these chairs can be great for some but not so good for others." He suggests giving one of these chairs as long a trial period as possible before deciding to buy.

Adjust your desk and work habits.

Working at a desk for extended periods can lead to back pain, and not just because of the sitting it requires: Movements such as bending over for files from a sitting position, holding a telephone pinched between the shoulder and ear, and working with the head tilted down-

* New York: Times Books, 1985.
† Toronto: McClelland and Stewart, 1987.

ward can take their toll even on a healthy spine, says Hage. He offers these tips for lightening the load of desk-bound endeavors.

■ Position your computer screen so that you are looking forward rather than downward when you work. According to the National Institute for Occupational Safety and Health, a computer keyboard should be placed 26 to 28 inches from the floor (the average desk is 30 to 32 inches high), and the screen should be angled so that the top of the screen is 10 degrees below eye level.

■ If your job involves reading and writing, raise your working surface to a comfortable level with what's called a slant board, an angled, adjustable surface with a ledge to keep books and papers in place. These are available in most art and drafting supply stores.

■ Use a speakerphone or a phone rest—a device that attaches to the receiver so the phone can be held without bending the neck—if you need to keep your hands free while phoning.

BACK TO SCHOOL

The prevalence of back pain in today's society has led to the development of the back school, a workshop or program designed to teach participants how to go about their daily activities while taking care of their backs. First implemented in Sweden at the Volvo automobile factory in the late 1960s, back schools are often found in the workplace to help reduce the risk (and costs) of on-the-job injuries.

These schools are legitimate and generally well regarded by the medical community. There are well over 1,000 back schools in the United States—one exists in most major American cities. They may be affiliated with a hospital, back-pain clinic, private practice or physician, or nonprofit group such as the YMCA. You can track down a back school in your area through the phone book or by asking your health-care practitioner for a referral.

Programs range from several hours to several weeks, and the prices vary accordingly. Check with your insurance company about reimbursement for the program—some plans may offer coverage, while others may not.

■ Do not lean over from your chair to access filing cabinets. Get up and access the cabinet by bending your knees while keeping your back straight.

■ Take breaks to walk around and stretch as often as possible.

Sleep on a back-friendly mattress.

In Chapter 2, we looked at the most back-friendly positions for sleeping, but what you sleep on can be just as important. Research indicates that a firm mattress does, in fact, tend to be best for preventing and relieving back pain in most people.

To test if this holds true for you, sleep on the floor on a makeshift mattress made of six to eight blankets, recommends Augustus A. White III, M.D., professor of orthopedic surgery at Harvard Medical School. If you feel better after three to five nights on this blanket bed, a firm mattress should be your choice. If not, opt for something softer.

Be sure to give your prospective purchase an adequate trial run in the store. Lie on the mattress for as long as your salesperson will allow and have your sleeping partner, if you have one, try it with you to see how it responds when he or she shifts or rolls over. The more "independence" the mattress allows, the better, White says.

And what about waterbeds? Again, let your comfort be your guide. Some back conditions are made better by sleeping on a waterbed, while others are made worse. Ask to sleep on one at a friend's house, rent one, or try one at a hotel.

Here are some other tips from White for maximizing your sleeping comfort.

■ Firm up your existing mattress by sliding a three-quarter-inch piece of plywood between it and your box spring. Any mattress that sags can be a back's worst nightmare.

■ Flip and rotate a new mattress every month for the first six months of use, and once every three months after that. This can prevent the development of uneven depressions in the mattress, which can make for uncomfortable sleep.

■ Treat yourself to a queen- or king-size mattress if you have a sleeping partner. You want your sleeping area to be as level and undisturbed as possible.

■ Request that your mattress be supported with a portable bed board if you find yourself confronted with an uncomfortably soft mattress while staying at a hotel or motel. Most public lodgings have these boards. However, don't hesitate to move your mattress to the floor if you can't get one.

■ Arrange your pillows so that your head is at a height that allows your neck to follow your spine in a straight, level line.

The Back-Friendly Lifestyle: Strategies for Everyday Tasks

Be kind to your back while driving.

You needn't motor across the country to know how hard on the back driving can be. The vibrations of driving aggravate the spinal discs and nerves of the back on a cellular level. Also, the positions in which we drive and the poorly designed seats on which we sit can be sources of discomfort. Most of the newer-model cars now have seats that provide good lower-back support (you should be able to notice an obvious protrusion that presses into your lower back when driving), but you may need to make some adaptations if your car is an older model that does not.

As when sitting in a chair that lacks good lumbar support, place a small pillow between the seat and the small of your back, and tighten your seat belt to keep your hips from sliding forward, recommends Edward A. Abraham, M.D., assistant clinical professor of orthopedics at the University of California, Irvine, in his book *Freedom From Back Pain*. Also, adjust your seat so that you're far enough forward to allow you to maintain an upright position while working the pedals. If you have to stretch to reach the pedals, you're apt to slide forward in your seat into a slouching position, which will increase pressure on your spine dramatically.

Follow these other tips for making driving less stressful to the back.

■ Take regular breaks when driving long distances. "Stop every hour or two to walk around the car and stretch," says Harris H. McIlwain, M.D., in his book *Winning With Back Pain*. In addition to helping decompress the spine from the pressures of sitting (giving a breather to spinal discs), this can help reoxygenate the muscles of the back, minimizing stiffness and fatigue. It also can give your back a break from the vibrations caused by driving.

■ Use your car's armrests to help lighten your back's load.

■ Tilt your rearview mirror slightly upward to encourage yourself to maintain a good, upright sitting position while driving.

■ Use cruise control if your car has it so that you can more easily shift positions to avoid stiffness when driving.

■ When you're getting out of a car, lift and swing both legs out of the door, place both feet on the ground, and then stand up, recommends an article in the April 1994 issue of *Prevention* magazine. This locks together the legs and the pelvis and forces you to turn on your buttocks. Setting one foot outside the door at a time forces your back to twist away from your hips, which can strain the back.

Think before you lift.

Lifting has the potential for putting more pressure on the spine than any other activity, so follow these dos and don'ts for safer lifting offered by the American Academy of Orthopaedic Surgeons and other back experts. And observe these tips when doing *any* lifting—from picking up a child to hauling a heavy suitcase—no matter how easy it may seem. Often it's the routine lifts we do that entail the greatest risk, back experts say, because we attempt them from the most potentially dangerous positions.

■ **Do** begin with a firm base, with your feet about shoulder-width apart.

■ **Don't** bend at the waist; lower yourself by bending at the knees, instead.

■ **Do** position yourself as close to the object you're lifting as possible, and hold the object as close to your body as possible once it's hoisted.

■ **Don't** twist as you lift: Your spinal discs will be under enough pressure as it is without having to endure the additional burden of rotation.

■ **Do** loosen up before lifting, by bending backward several times with your hands on your hips.

■ **Don't** lift when wearing shoes with high heels.

■ **Do** help support your spine by tightening your stomach muscles as you lift.

■ **Don't** ever lean over something to make a lift, such as over a piece of furniture to open a window.

■ **Do** be certain to have secure footing before attempting a lift so you don't slip, and be sure the path ahead of you is clear if you're going to be carrying something for a distance.

■ **Don't** lift anything heavy over your head.

■ **Do** avoid lifting any object whose size makes it awkward, even if it's not heavy.

■ **Don't** keep trying to lift an object if you experience any discomfort. Even if the pain is minor, it very quickly could become major if you try to work through it.

Information about safe lifting practices in the workplace is available from the National Institute for Occupational Safety and Health (NIOSH). You can contact NIOSH at 4676 Columbia Parkway, Cincinnati, OH 45226-1998; 800-35-NIOSH.

Use back-friendly tools and gadgets.

More and more, technology is coming to the rescue of those with back pain by creating helpful gizmos to take the pressure off—why not take advantage of them? For especially back-taxing chores such as shoveling snow, raking leaves, mopping the kitchen floor, and digging in the garden, you can make life easier on your back in several ways.

A number of items have been specially designed with "gooseneck" handles and other features to minimize the bending and lifting that make these jobs so tough on the back. Even a tool as simple as a shoehorn–which saves you from having to bend over to pull your shoes on–can help save you from back troubles.

For more information on back-saving tools, check out your local hardware store, visit the gadget store at the mall, or contact Comfortably Yours, 52 Hunter Avenue, Maywood, NJ 07607; 201-368-0400.

Use back-saving form when shoveling or raking.

It's important to use proper form when shoveling and raking. When shoveling, follow this advice.

- Bend your legs, not your back.
- Keep the shovel as close to your body as possible.
- Keep the size and weight of each shovel load modest.
- Take frequent rests to prevent excessive fatigue.

When raking, use this form.

- Keep your knees slightly bent.
- Position one foot slightly out in front of the other.
- Keep your rake close to your body to avoid excessive leaning or stretching.

Keep your back properly dressed in cold weather.

Cold weather can increase the likelihood of muscle spasms when you are working or playing outdoors, so dress with your back in mind.

- Make sure your shirt is long enough that it doesn't expose your back by coming untucked.
- Dress in layers so you can dress down to prevent excessive sweating.
- Wear a "wick-through" fabric (such as Thinsulate) directly against

your skin so that perspiration will be pulled into your outer layers of clothing, preventing chilling.

Flatten your wallet.

According to Augustus A. White III, M.D., professor of orthopedic surgery at Harvard Medical School, in his book *Your Aching Back*, a patient who had been suffering from hip and leg pain experienced total relief when the source of his back pain was discovered. The cause? Impingement of his sciatic nerve by the inch-and-a-half-thick wallet in the rear pocket of his pants that he sat on when he drove. Be careful to keep similarly bulky items out of your trouser back pockets.

The Mind-Body Connection: Using Relaxation Techniques

Reduce stress.

In much the same way that stress can precipitate headaches, it can contribute to back pain: Tense thoughts can produce tense muscles, and tense muscles can produce pain. "A person with low-back pain who is emotionally upset or stressed will often be very tense . . . which causes the muscles to tighten even more," notes an official statement by the American Academy of Orthopaedic Surgery.

Some experts believe, too, that stress is one of the leading causes of back pain. John Sarno, M.D., a physiatrist at New York University's Rusk Institute of Rehabilitation Medicine, believes that back pain comes from muscle spasms produced by tension more than 95 percent of the time.

If you suspect that your back pain may be related to emotional stress in your life, your first course of action should be to try to identify and then eliminate the source of that stress. Whether you're dissatisfied with your job, unhappy with a relationship, or simply feeling swamped by responsibilities, your vulnerability to back pain probably will continue until you resolve the cause of your stress.

For anxieties that are less deep-seated, however–the occasional traffic jam, family problem, or "killer" day at your job–simply taking time out to achieve a state of deep relaxation often can help, says cardiologist Herbert Benson, M.D., chief of the division of behavioral medicine at New England Deaconess Hospital in Boston and associate professor of medicine at Harvard Medical School, in his book *The Relaxation Response*.* Various strategies such as biofeedback, meditation, self-hypnosis, and visualization therapy (see box) can be employed to achieve this state of therapeutic calmness, which Benson calls the relaxation response. But just as effective can be this simpler technique Benson has developed based on his recent studies at Harvard. It's essentially a distillation of the more elaborate disciplines mentioned above, but it can produce similar results, Benson says, if practiced with commitment and focus.

For best results in preventing backache, try to practice the technique regularly for 10 to 20 minutes at least twice a day, Benson says. The technique also can be used on an as-needed basis to relieve a case of stress-induced back pain that has come on suddenly. Here's how to do it.

■ Sit comfortably with your eyes closed.

■ Choose a word or phrase that has a pleasant and personal meaning to you (the name of a loved one or special place or a lyric from a favorite song, for example).

■ Consciously relax your entire body.

■ Begin to breathe deeply and slowly, silently repeating your word or phrase to yourself each time you exhale.

■ Try not to focus on any particular thoughts that may come into your mind. Instead, acknowledge them and let them drift away.

■ Continue in this relaxed and passive state for 10 to 20 minutes.

Make peace at work.

Yes, many of us have jobs that can give us pains in our backs, says Stanley J. Bigos, M.D., founder and director of the Spine Resource

* New York: Avon, 1976.

RELAXATION STRATEGIES

Stress can bring on or exacerbate pain, making relaxation one of the keys to preventing backache. A number of strategies can be employed to help take away tension and achieve the relaxation response. Here is a brief rundown of some of the most well-known paths to relaxed muscles, a calm attitude, and reduced stress.

■ **Aromatherapy.** This strategy involves the inhalation or application of fragrant oils to promote relaxation. Scents can be released through candles, lotions, massage oils, and perfumes, or oils may be added to a warm bath.

■ **Biofeedback.** Also a means of treating back pain, this technique involves concentration to control usually unconscious functions, such as heart rate and body temperature, to reduce muscle tension. It is taught by using electronic monitoring of the body's responses.

■ **Deep breathing.** Relaxation is promoted by concentrating on taking slow, rhythmic breaths. This technique often is used in combination with other stress-reducing methods.

■ **Hydrotherapy.** This method relies on the use of water, in the form of bathing, swimming, or using a sauna or whirlpool, to heal and relax. This technique also is used as a therapy for back pain.

■ **Meditation.** Relaxation is promoted by concentrating on one object or word (called a mantra) while ignoring all external stimuli.

■ **Progressive muscle relaxation.** This technique involves systematically contracting and relaxing the muscles in order from the toes to the head to promote relaxation.

■ **Self-hypnosis.** In this strategy, a person uses specific mental commands to self-induce a light hypnotic trance, promoting relaxation and restoration.

■ **Visualization therapy.** This method involves visualizing a pleasant situation or imagining the departure of any stressors to promote relaxation.

Clinic in Seattle and professor of orthopedic surgery and environmental health at the University of Washington School of Medicine, based on a study of more than 3,000 employees of the Boeing Company. In the study, done by the Spine Resource Clinic, workers who said they "hardly ever" enjoyed their jobs were found to be more than twice as likely to suffer from back pain as workers who said they "almost always" enjoyed their work. Upon closer inspection of the survey results, Bigos found that "the job itself does not seem to matter as much as how well you get along with your supervisor."

There are some steps you can take to try to come to terms with an unsatisfying job. If you're unhappy with your supervisor, make an appointment to discuss the reasons for your dissatisfaction, and be open-minded about what emerges from that meeting. Try to improve your situation by communicating with coworkers and participating in the office environment. Attend meetings, express your feelings, and get feedback from those around you. As a last resort, consider asking to be transferred to a different department with a new supervisor, or to another type of job for which you might be better suited.

If you're resigned to the fact that you're in the wrong position, put your energies into the positive activity of finding another place of employment. Maybe you need additional knowledge or skills that could be acquired through workshops, night courses, or books your supervisor might recommend.

4 The Future of Back Care

Despite the fact that back pain affects more than 80 percent of the population at some point in their lives—and the fact that $70 billion is spent each year on back pain—medical science is far from developing foolproof methods to diagnose and treat back pain. Unlike with smallpox and polio, a vaccine for backache will never be found, and it's unlikely that a medication or surgical technique will surface to cure sufferers once and for all.

But even though the complexities of the back and the myriad factors that contribute to pain may preclude a definitive backache cure, experts in the field are still envisioning—and working toward—that elusive goal. Here, several well-known back-pain experts explain the paths they believe may lead us to a pain-free future.

New Angles on Prevention

Of course, the best way to end our struggle with back pain is to prevent it from occurring in the first place, says Stanley J. Bigos, M.D., founder and director of the Spine Resource Clinic in Seattle and professor of orthopedic surgery and environmental health at the University of Washington School of Medicine.

"There's no small irony in that the country with the most advanced health-care system in the world also suffers from the most back pain in the world," Bigos says. "We would do far better in the future to increase our efforts at preventing back pain from progressing to the point of needing our elaborate treatments in the first place. . . . More and more, we're learning that back pain is a condition where prevention is worth not a pound of cure but rather something closer to a ton."

What Bigos hopes will be impressed on future generations is that exercise is the cornerstone of any back-pain prevention program. "Back pain is not so much a problem of wear and tear as it is one of waste due to neglect," he says. More attention also needs to be given to factors that precipitate back pain in the workplace and to how psychological issues such as stress affect back pain, he says.

To this end, Bigos hopes to see proper back care taught in the schools–possibly as early as grade school–right along with other health basics such as proper hygiene and nutrition. In fact, educators in Great Britain have already begun to implement such programs. "In general, we as doctors need to impress on our patients that their backs are their responsibilities far more so than ours, and this applies to every aspect of their lives," says Bigos.

Even though doctors are beginning to learn the importance of self-care in the prevention and treatment of back pain, many are slow to move toward the role of patient educator. However, according to Charles V. Burton, M.D., medical director of the Institute for Low Back Pain Care in Minneapolis and coauthor of *Managing Low Back Pain*, the new wave of back-pain treatment will be one of "total care," meaning doctors will be encouraged to carry treatment far beyond a patient's medical treatment program.*

In the future, Burton says, practitioners not only will diagnose and treat patients from a medical standpoint but also will educate their patients on what they can do for themselves to keep their backs healthy even after they've recovered. "We must influence patients to take responsibility for themselves, and we must give them the information they need to do so," he says.

William H. Kirkaldy-Willis, M.D., who coauthored *Managing Low Back Pain* with Burton, agrees that doctors must learn to get their patients involved in their own care. Kirkaldy-Willis, professor of orthopedic surgery at the University of Saskatchewan, believes that "greater patient participation," inspired by physicians, will be the primary thrust of back care in the years to come. "In the early stages of back pain,

---

* New York: Churchill Livingstone, 1992.

especially, we need to put more effort into guiding patients toward things they can do for themselves," he says.

But this guidance must be more than purely physical, Kirkaldy-Willis adds. "In helping an individual back to health, we need to think of the whole person," he says. This means addressing a patient's emotional and even spiritual components. "Often we can help the physical components of a patient's problem by treating the emotional ones, and vice versa. We need to be more aware of this interconnection, and use it," says Kirkaldy-Willis.

Partnerships for Better Back Health

Most likely, your relationship with your practitioner ends as soon as you leave the office—usually after a visit of only a few minutes. But Kirkaldy-Willis believes that will change in the years to come. "Greater benefits can be obtained when the health-care practitioner works right alongside the patient," he says. And when he says "right alongside," he means the doctor or physical therapist working out on the treadmill next to yours at the gym.

One such aggressive hands-on approach is already in place at the Back-In-Action Clinic directed by Roy Slack, M.D., in Lake Oswega, Oregon. The program is one of tough, progressive therapeutic exercises. At the clinic, therapists often work directly alongside patients, doing the same exercises while encouraging patients and spurring them on. Slack reports that this working together of patient and therapist is extremely effective. The success rate at the clinic, which deals primarily with the most dire cases of back pain, runs at an impressive 84 percent. The success of Slack's approach has led to the establishment of similar clinics throughout the United States.

Also encouraging have been recent efforts by some back-care clinics to align themselves with commercial fitness centers so that patients can do their rehabilitative exercises in a more communal and less "medicinal" environment, reports Steve Burns, D.C., of the Fourth Avenue Chiropractic Clinic in Saskatoon, Saskatchewan.

"This approach has a number of attractive features," Burns explains. "The fitness center is already in operation, so the cost per patient is nominal—usually only between $50 and $100 [for a six-week program].

"The center also has a health-oriented atmosphere where participants are referred to as clients or members rather than patients. Participants in such programs, consequently, gain a greater sense of responsibility and control over their conditions than they would in a more clinical setting."

Many participants enjoy their experiences so much that they choose to remain as club members when their rehabilitations are complete, Burns says. This is important because failure to keep patients in shape is one of the most common reasons back-care programs fail, he adds.

Advancements in Technology

You may already be accustomed to stopping at your drugstore's computerized blood-pressure cuff for a quick check. Efforts are now underway to give the computer an increasingly important role in helping us to "doctor" ourselves, says Malcolm H. Pope, Dr.Med.Sc., Ph.D., director of the Iowa Spine Research Center and professor of biomedical engineering at the University of Iowa. "The more we can involve people in their own treatment, the more success against back pain we're going to have, and the computer offers great potential for helping us do this," Pope says.

The computerized system proposed by P. Thomas Davis, D.C., of the Center for Clinical Studies at the Northwestern College of Chiropractic in Minneapolis, would have back-pain sufferers fill out a computerized questionnaire asking about symptoms they are experiencing as well as their medical histories and lifestyles. The computer would then process this information and come up with a treatment program that would include, for example, daily exercises and suggestions for safeguarding the back while at home and work. Ideally, the service would be available in public places such as shopping malls and grocery stores.

"The clientele for such a system would be anyone with back pain or an allied musculoskeletal condition that was causing sufficient discomfort to need help, but not so much that it seemed necessary to consult a medical expert," Davis says. Only if the treatment program failed to bring relief would the patient be advised to seek additional medical treatment.

Technology has also brightened the future for those with back pain that requires surgery. Progress in the medical treatment of back pain will continue to be made, says Burton. Efforts will continue toward the development of artificial discs to replace those that have ruptured or degenerated. In addition, new fusing techniques are being developed to treat those whose spines are unstable. These techniques use flexible, nonmetallic rods rather than bone grafting to fuse the spine.

Also, the minimally invasive surgical techniques such as microsurgery that are available today will continue to be refined in the future. The primary advantage of less invasive surgery over more traditional, open surgery (in which the spinal column and spinal cord are exposed) is faster recovery, explain Richard Fraser, M.D., professor of neurosurgery at Cornell University Medical College, and Ann Forer in their book *The Well-Informed Patient's Guide to Back Surgery*.* The new techniques involve less disruption of the muscles, ligaments, and tendons that surround the spinal cord than open surgery does.

In microsurgery, incisions of only one-half inch are required, and the work is performed with tiny instruments. The surgeons are aided by microscopes fed into the area of operation via a flexible tube. In many cases, only local anesthesia is required, and patients often are permitted to return home the same day surgery is performed. This usually allows for a full recovery within weeks (and in some cases, even days) rather than the months required with more traditional surgical techniques.

Back-Care Research

Much of how we treat back pain in the future will rely on what we discover about back pain in the present. Professor of orthopedic surgery at Harvard Medical School and author of *Your Aching Back* Augustus A. White III, M.D., maintains that back pain is such an intricate physiological as well as psychological problem that in many ways we've just begun to scratch the surface in understanding it.†

---

* New York: Dell, 1992.
† New York: Simon and Schuster, 1990.

White predicts that new research on the prevention, diagnosis, and treatment of back pain will open doors for those working toward the end of back pain. In White's vision of the future, experts have unraveled mysteries such as the relationship between emotional stress and back pain; the role hereditary conditions such as scoliosis play in chronic back pain; and the link between hormonal changes, nutrition, lifestyle choices, and back problems. White hopes that with this research, experts will be able to determine who is at high risk for back pain.

Refined diagnostic and treatment methods also will be available. According to White, back-pain sufferers may look forward to innovations such as an MRI (magnetic resonance imaging) system that can evaluate the spine while it is in motion; several types of new drugs that work on the central nervous system to block pain, that work directly on the injured area to reduce inflammation, and that treat back pain linked to stress by improving mood; and, of course, advanced surgical techniques such as those discussed above.

White also expects that employers and corporations will take more responsibility for back pain, creating products and policies that make things easier on the back. For example, we may look forward to orthopedically correct seat designs in cars, airplanes, and public transportation, White says. Additionally, those who suffer from back pain may also enjoy an improved system of financial compensation. "Our current system too often works in ways that perpetuate pain behavior and disability," White says. "In the future, we can look forward to a rewriting of the compensation laws so that justice is assured to the individual back-pain sufferer as well as to society."

GLOSSARY

Acupressure: A system of massage inherited from the Orient that seeks to relieve pain and promote healing by applying manual pressure to key pathways called meridians.

Acupuncture: An ancient Chinese art of healing and pain relief whereby thin needles are inserted just under the skin into key pathways called meridians

Acute: A term describing an attack of sharp, intense pain that tends to be short in duration.

Allopathic physician: A traditional medical doctor who holds the degree of doctor of medicine (M.D.). Allopaths focus on finding the cause and nature of a disease or a condition, then counter that condition using therapy, medications, or surgery.

Ankylosing spondylitis: A form of arthritis in which the vertebrae of the spine become fused due to the development of bony growths.

Antidepressants: A category of medications used to treat nerve-associated pain, insomnia, and depression related to backache. They include imipramine and trazodone.

Arthritis: Chronic inflammation and irritation within joints characterized by stiffness and pain, especially after periods of immobility such as bed rest or prolonged sitting. There are more than 200 different types of arthritis, including osteoarthritis, rheumatoid arthritis, and ankylosing spondylitis.

Benign: A term used to describe a growth that is noncancerous and poses no biological threat to neighboring tissue.

Biofeedback: A process in which an individual monitors (usually electronically) one or more physiological systems (such as heart rate, blood pressure, or muscle tension) in order to learn how to gain voluntary control of that system.

Biopsy: The removal of a sample of bodily tissue for the purpose of microscopic examination.

Bone scan: A diagnostic procedure in which a radioactive substance that adheres to bone is injected into the system and visualized with an imaging device. It is used to diagnose abnormalities such as fractures, infections, and bone degeneration.

Cartilage: A form of connective tissue that acts as a cushioning device where bones meet within joints.

Cervical vertebrae: The seven topmost vertebrae between the base of the skull and the chest that comprise the neck. The term "cervical" describes the upper back and spine.

Chiropractic therapy: A system of spinal care based on the theory that most back problems, and many health complications in general, are due to misalignment of spinal vertebrae. A practitioner who practices chiropractic therapy holds a degree of doctor of chiropractic, or D.C.

Chronic: A term describing attacks of pain or disease that tend to be long-lasting and/or recurrent on a regular basis.

Coccyx: The four semifused segments at the lower end of the spine, also known as the tailbone. Pain in this region is known as coccygodynia.

Collagen: A protein formed by the body as a major component of ligaments, tendons, scar tissue, and bone.

Complementary therapies: Nontraditional approaches to treating back pain (such as acupressure, biofeedback, relaxation techniques, and yoga) that seek to restore health by achieving harmony between the emotional as well as physical aspects of the body. They are considered complementary because they are often used in conjunction with traditional therapies.

Compression: Pressure on the spine created by deterioration of vertebrae due to fractures or natural wear. It can result in painful pressure on a nerve root.

Computerized tomography (CT scan): A type of x-ray that uses computers to create three-dimensional images of bone and soft tissue that can be seen on several planes at once.

Connective tissues: Tissues (such as ligaments and tendons) that serve to hold together body structures, such as muscle fibers and bone.

Corticosteroid: A type of medication used for short periods usually to reduce acute inflammation within joints.

Counterirritant: A therapy or medication that relieves pain by stimulating the nerves in the affected area with a lesser pain or irritation. The stimulation serves to "distract" the mind from the greater pain.

Disc degeneration: Changes in spinal discs resulting in loss of elasticity and volume and, hence, a narrowing of the space between vertebral bodies.

Discography: A diagnostic test in which dye is injected into the spinal column in order to diagnose an abnormal or degenerating disc. It is also called myelography.

Electrophysiologic tests: Diagnostic tests that assess muscular activity by measuring how fast the muscles transmit electrical nerve impulses.

Ergonomics: The study of bodily movement for the purpose of designing optimally safe and effective facilities and equipment for both work and recreational activities.

Facet joints: The sites at which the vertebrae interlock at the rear of the spine.

Fusion: An surgical operation that permanently bonds vertebrae for the purpose of eliminating motion of the joints and stabilizing the spine.

Gout: A form of arthritis caused by a buildup of uric acid in the body.

Herniated (or **ruptured) disc:** The displacement of the material contained in the soft center of the spinal disc beyond its normal confines.

Hydrotherapy: A therapy that uses water in a liquid, solid, or gaseous form to treat backache and promote relaxation. Icing a sore muscle, taking a hot shower, using a humidifier, and swimming are all forms of hydrotherapy.

Hyperkyphosis: An abnormally accentuated curvature of the middle (thoracic) region of the spine.

Hyperlordosis: An abnormally accentuated curvature in the lower (lumbar) region of the spine.

Idiopathic: Having no known cause.

Ligament: A strand of dense connective tissue that holds bones together to form joints.

Lumbago: An antiquated term referring to back pain in general.

Lumbar vertebrae: The five vertebrae located at the base of the back, above the coccyx, or tailbone. The term "lumbar" refers to the lower back.

Magnetic resonance imaging (MRI): A diagnostic technique that employs a superconducting magnet plus a computer to create precise images of soft tissue (such as muscles, ligaments, tendons, and tumors) within the body.

Malignant: Referring to a cancerous growth that tends to spread throughout the body with destructive results to other tissues and organs.

Massage therapy: A manual therapy used to promote healing by improving circulation, easing muscle tension, and encouraging relaxation.

Meningitis: A potentially fatal infection of the meninges, the protective membranes that cover the brain and the spinal cord.

Metastasize: To spread to other parts of the body, as in the transfer of the cancerous cells of a malignant tumor through the lymph system or bloodstream to a new location in the body.

Microsurgery: Minimally invasive surgery, performed with the aid of a microscope, that greatly reduces damage to muscles and other tissues in the surgical area.

Muscle relaxants: Drugs used to relieve pain caused by muscular tension. Muscle relaxants include those from the class of drugs known as benzodiazepines (Librium, Valium, Xanax) and sedative medications.

Neurologist: A medical doctor who specializes in diagnosing and treating problems associated with the nervous system.

Neuropathy: Any disease involving the nerves. The prefix "neuro" refers to the body's nervous system.

Neurosurgeon: A medical doctor who specializes in the surgical treatment of disorders of the brain, spinal cord, and nerves.

Nonsteroidal anti-inflammatory drugs (NSAIDs): Drugs, other than steroids, used to reduce inflammation within tissue. NSAIDs include aspirin and ibuprofen.

Orthopedics: The medical specialty that deals with the treatment and prevention of disorders of the musculoskeletal system, including the bones, muscles, ligaments, tendons, and joints. Orthopedists and orthopedic surgeons are the professionals who specialize in orthopedics.

Osteoarthritis: A form of arthritis that involves deterioration of the cartilage and other lubricating tissues within the joints responsible for keeping the joints moving freely.

Osteopathy: A medical discipline that concentrates on treating the body as a whole, focusing on the body's joints, muscles, bones, ligaments, and tendons in particular. An osteopathic physician holds a degree of doctor of osteopathy (D.O.) rather than the degree doctor of medicine (M.D.) held by the allopathic physician. D.O.'s are more likely to perform spinal manipulation and other manual therapies than M.D.'s but are otherwise similar.

Osteophytes (also called **bone spurs):** Bony growths that frequently form on vertebrae in response to irritation caused by disc degeneration, but which also can develop due to natural wear and tear.

Paget's disease: A condition characterized by painful enlargement of the bones frequently involving the vertebrae of the lumbar spine.

Physiatrist: A physician who specializes in treating musculoskeletal problems primarily through rehabilitative exercise and deep massage.

Physical therapist: A person trained to treat patients through physical means such as heat, massage, and exercise.

Referred pain: Pain experienced at a site other than where it originates. For example, pressure on a nerve in the spinal column may result in referred pain in the buttocks.

Relaxin: A hormone produced during the later stages of pregnancy that can contribute to back pain by causing the ligaments of the pelvis and lumbar spine to relax, thus reducing the spine's ability to retain its normal posture.

Rheumatoid arthritis: A form of arthritis that involves chronic inflammation of joints and connective tissue throughout the body. It is frequently accompanied by fatigue and loss of appetite in addition to the common arthritis symptoms.

Rheumatologist: A physician specializing in the treatment of arthritis.

Sacrum: The wedge-shaped bone, created by the fusion of five vertebrae, at the back of the pelvis, above the coccyx. The sacrum supports the lumbar vertebrae.

Sciatica: Pain extending along the path of the sciatic nerve, which runs over the buttocks and down the outside of the leg to the toes.

Scoliosis: A progressive, abnormal lateral curve of the thoracic or lumbar spine.

Shiatsu: A Japanese form of acupressure that uses finger pressure to massage key pathways called meridians.

Spasm: A sudden, painful contraction of muscle fibers that occurs involuntarily and often persists.

Spinal cord: An extension of the brain through which nerve impulses travel. The spinal cord extends through, and is protected by, the vertebrae.

Spinal discs: Fibrous pads with soft, gel-like centers that are located between the vertebrae to provide cushioning.

Spinal manipulation: A technique employed primarily by chiropractors, but also osteopaths and some physical therapists, in which a twisting or stretching action is used to align spinal vertebrae and to provide movement between facet joints that have become fixated due to muscle spasm or injury.

Spinal nerves: The 31 pairs of nerves branching out from the spinal cord that transmit and receive nerve impulses from all areas of the body.

Spinal stenosis: An abnormal narrowing of the spinal canal resulting in damaging pressure on the spinal nerves.

Spondylolisthesis: An unhealed fracture across the back of one of the vertebrae of the spine (usually inherited), which tends to make the spine unstable.

Spondylolysis: A condition of the spine characterized by osteophytes (bony growths), thickening of the bones of the vertebrae, and degeneration of spinal discs.

Sprain: A tearing of a ligament.

Steroids: A group of drugs, which includes cortisone, that reduces inflammation. They are sometimes used to treat back pain on a short-term basis.

Strain: The overstretching of a muscle.

Synovial fluid: The lubricating fluid contained within joints.

Synovial membrane: The delicate membrane that lines the inside of a joint. Inflammation of a synovial membrane is known as synovitis.

Swayback: An exaggerated forward curvature of the lumbar spine.

Tendinitis: Inflammation of a tendon.

Tendon: Connective tissue that connects muscle fibers to bone.

Thermography: A diagnostic technique that detects abnormalities in the body by measuring variations in temperatures throughout the body.

Thoracic vertebrae: The 12 spinal vertebrae of the upper back corresponding to the 12 ribs of the thorax (chest). The term "thoracic" refers to the midback area.

Transcutaneous electrical nerve stimulation (TENS): The delivery of brief pulses of mild electrical current through the skin for the purpose of relieving pain within underlying nerve fibers.

Trigger point: An area of localized tenderness within a muscle thought to be the result of long-standing pain being referred from elsewhere in the body.

Ultrasound: A therapy that involves the use of sound vibrations to relieve muscular pain and stiffness.

Vertebrae: The 24 bony segments of the spine. They are also known as vertebral bodies.

Vertebral canal: The tunnel created by the vertebrae of the spine through which the spinal cord and spinal nerves pass.

Whiplash: Injury to ligaments of the neck resulting usually from a sudden backward movement of the head.

X-ray: A diagnostic technique which employs electromagnetic radiation to produce images of the bones and other opaque structures within the body.

Yoga: A discipline that seeks to unite mind and body through postures, stretches, and breathing techniques designed to dissipate emotional and physical stress.

INDEX

D

E

F

G

H

T

U

V

W

X

Y